The Balanced LOW POTASSIUM COOKBOOK

Wholesome, Low-Sodium Meals to Help Manage Kidney Disease, Balance Blood Pressure, and Support Heart Health

OPAL HENSLEY

Copyright © 2025 by Opal Hensley

All rights reserved.

No part of this publication may be reproduced, distributed, or transmitted in any form or by any means, including photocopying, recording, or other electronic or mechanical methods, without the prior written permission of the author, except in the case of brief quotations embodied in critical reviews and certain other noncommercial uses permitted by copyright law.

Disclaimer:

The content of this book is not intended to be a substitute for professional medical advice, diagnosis, or treatment. Always seek the advice of your physician or other qualified health providers with any questions you may have regarding a medical condition. Never disregard professional medical advice or delay in seeking it because of something you have read in this book.

Table of Contents

Introduction 4
   Understanding Potassium and Its Role in the Body 5
   What Is Hyperkalemia? 7
   The Importance of a Low-Potassium Diet 9
   Identifying High and Low Potassium Foods 11
   Tips for Reading Nutrition Labels 14

Chapter 1: Breakfast Delights 16
   Herbed Egg White Omelet 17
   Blueberry Pancakes with Maple Syrup 19
   Creamy Rice Porridge with Apples 21
   Low-Potassium Smoothie Bowl 23
   Oatmeal with Cinnamon and Pears 25
   Banana-Free Breakfast Muffins 27
   Applesauce Pancakes with Agave 29
   Low-Potassium Granola Parfait 31
   Scrambled Tofu with Bell Peppers 33
   Rye Toast with Cream Cheese and Strawberries 35

Chapter 2: Wholesome Lunches 36
   Grilled Chicken Salad with Cranberries 37
   Turkey and Cucumber Sandwich 39
   Quinoa Salad with Roasted Vegetables 41
   Low-Potassium Lentil Soup 43
   Stuffed Bell Peppers with Ground Turkey 45
   Egg Salad Lettuce Wraps 47
   Rice Noodle Bowl with Fresh Herbs 49
   Chicken and Apple Slaw Wrap 51
   Tuna Salad on White Bread 53
   Couscous Bowl with Zucchini and Carrots 54

Chapter 3: Satisfying Dinners 56

Baked Cod with Lemon and Herbs 57

Grilled Pork Chops with Apple Chutney 59

Stir-Fried Rice with Mixed Vegetables 61

Roasted Chicken with Garlic and Rosemary 63

Beef Stir-Fry with Snow Peas 64

Turkey Meatballs with Low-Potassium Marinara 66

Ginger-Honey Glazed Salmon 67

Chicken Stir-Fry with Bok Choy 68

Baked Ziti with Low-Potassium Cheese 69

Sweet and Sour Chicken with Rice 71

Chapter 4: Kidney-Friendly Snacks 73

Cucumber and Cream Cheese Bites 74

Rice Cakes with Honey Drizzle 75

Unsalted Pretzel Mix 76

Apple Slices with Almond Butter 77

Homemade Popcorn with Herbs 78

Chapter 5: Desserts and Sweet Treats 79

Vanilla Pudding with Berries 80

Lemon Sorbet 81

Rice Pudding with Cinnamon 82

Angel Food Cake with Strawberries 83

Low-Potassium Fruit Salad 84

Chapter 7: 30-Day Meal Plan 85

Week 1: Getting Started 85

Week 2: Building Momentum 87

Week 3: Exploring New Flavors 89

Week 4: Maintaining the Lifestyle 91

Meal Prep Tips for a Low-Potassium Lifestyle 93

Conclusion: A Final Note 95

Introduction

This cookbook is written for anyone who has been advised by a healthcare provider to follow a low-potassium diet. Whether you have compromised kidney function, are recovering from an illness, or simply want to prevent complications from excess potassium intake, The Balanced Low Potassium Cookbook is your go-to resource. It offers not only practical dietary guidance but also creative, flavorful, and nutrient-balanced recipes that do not compromise on taste or satisfaction.

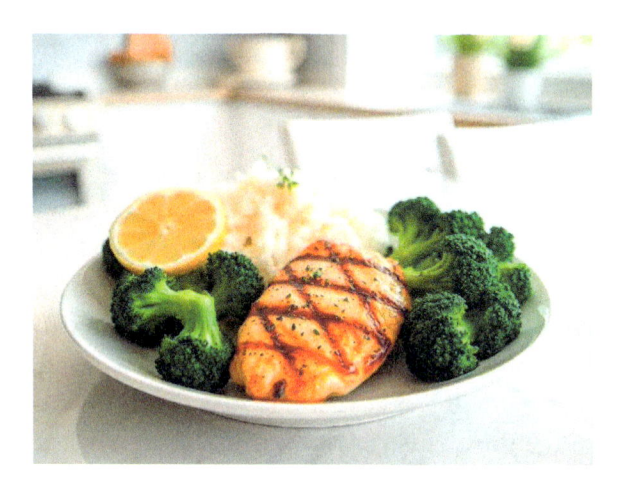

Why Potassium Becomes a Problem

Under normal circumstances, the kidneys maintain a healthy potassium balance by excreting excess amounts through urine. When kidney function is impaired, potassium builds up in the bloodstream. The higher the level, the more dangerous it becomes. For people living with kidney disease, careful dietary planning becomes as important as medical treatment. But potassium doesn't only come from obvious sources like bananas and potatoes—it's also hidden in common foods such as tomato sauces, beans, dairy products, chocolate, and certain whole grains.

One of the greatest challenges in adopting a low-potassium diet is understanding what foods to limit, avoid, or substitute. Even healthy foods can be problematic when potassium levels are not regulated. This book was developed to address those challenges with clarity, precision, and creativity. We understand that food is not only fuel—it is also comfort, tradition, and pleasure. Our mission is to ensure that a low-potassium diet can still be deeply enjoyable and culturally inclusive.

What You Will Find in This Book

This cookbook includes more than 40 carefully tested recipes, each created to be low in potassium without sacrificing flavor or nutrition. From savory breakfasts and satisfying lunches to comforting dinners and sweet treats, there's something for every taste and dietary need. Every recipe includes portion sizes, nutrition facts, and simple cooking instructions to make meal preparation easy, even for those with limited time or culinary experience.

Additionally, we've included a comprehensive 30-day meal plan tailored to meet the needs of individuals following a low-potassium regimen. This plan is designed to provide structure and variety while ensuring nutritional balance. You'll find grocery shopping guides, prep tips, and ingredient substitution ideas to help streamline your planning process.

Beyond recipes, the book also offers:

- An overview of potassium's role in the body
- A list of high- and low-potassium foods
- Tools for label reading and ingredient analysis
- Tips for managing potassium intake when dining out
- A guide for balancing fluid, sodium, and phosphorus levels, as these often go hand-in-hand with potassium management in chronic kidney disease

How to Use This Cookbook

The key to success with a low-potassium diet lies in planning, preparation, and consistency. While it may feel overwhelming at first, this book is structured to be both educational and practical. Each chapter builds upon the next, helping you gradually become more confident in making informed food choices. You are encouraged to adapt the recipes to suit your specific preferences, allergies, or medical advice from your healthcare provider or dietitian.

Whether you are new to this lifestyle or looking to expand your recipe collection, this cookbook is designed to empower you. You will learn to identify safe foods, cook with confidence, and bring joy back into your kitchen. Your health journey is unique, but you do not have to walk it alone. With this guide, you'll discover that eating for health can also mean eating with delight.

Understanding Potassium and Its Role in the Body

Potassium is one of the most important minerals in the human body. It is classified as an electrolyte, a substance that conducts electricity when dissolved in water, which is essential for many physiological processes. Alongside sodium, calcium, chloride, and magnesium, potassium plays a central role in maintaining the balance of fluids and supporting the proper function of cells, tissues, and organs.

The average adult body contains about 3,500 to 4,500 milligrams of potassium per day, most of which is stored inside the cells. Despite its abundance, even small imbalances in potassium levels can have significant consequences. That's why potassium levels in the blood are tightly regulated, typically maintained between 3.5 and 5.0 milliequivalents per liter (mEq/L).

The Key Roles of Potassium

Regulating Heart Function: Potassium is crucial for maintaining a healthy heartbeat. It works in tandem with other electrolytes to transmit electrical signals that prompt the heart to contract and relax. A deficiency (hypokalemia) or excess (hyperkalemia) of potassium can disrupt these signals and result in dangerous arrhythmias.

- **Muscle Contraction:** All muscles—including the heart and skeletal muscles require potassium to contract properly. When potassium levels are off balance, it can lead to muscle weakness, cramps, twitching, or even paralysis in severe cases.

- Nerve Transmission: Potassium supports the transmission of electrical signals in the nervous system. It helps generate the action potentials that carry signals along neurons, enabling communication between the brain, spinal cord, and the rest of the body.

- Fluid and Electrolyte Balance: Potassium works with sodium to maintain fluid balance at the cellular level. Sodium draws fluid into cells, while potassium helps expel it. This delicate push-pull mechanism supports blood pressure regulation and ensures cells do not shrink or swell excessively.

- Kidney Function: The kidneys play a major role in controlling potassium levels. They filter excess potassium from the blood and excrete it in urine. In individuals with compromised kidney function, potassium may accumulate in the bloodstream, leading to hyperkalemia.

Dietary Sources of Potassium

Potassium is naturally abundant in many foods, particularly whole and unprocessed items. Fruits and vegetables are especially rich in potassium—bananas, oranges, tomatoes, potatoes, and leafy greens being among the top sources. Legumes, dairy products, nuts, and whole grains also contribute significantly to daily potassium intake.

In fact, the average adult consumes 2,500 to 4,700 mg of potassium per day, which aligns with general dietary recommendations. However, for individuals who must follow a low-potassium diet, the target intake is significantly lower—usually between 1,500 and 2,000 mg per day. The exact number should always be guided by a healthcare provider based on individual health status.

Why Potassium Becomes a Concern

Potassium levels in the body are maintained through a balance of dietary intake, kidney function, and cellular storage. When one of these components is impaired, potassium can accumulate in the blood. People with chronic kidney disease (CKD) are particularly at risk because their kidneys cannot excrete excess potassium efficiently.

Other risk factors include:

- Certain medications (e.g., ACE inhibitors, potassium-sparing diuretics)
- Addison's disease (adrenal insufficiency)
- Uncontrolled diabetes
- Severe infections, trauma, or burns
- Dehydration or severe bleeding

Symptoms of Potassium Imbalance

Most people don't feel symptoms of mild potassium imbalance. However, as levels become too high or too low, symptoms may include:

- Heart palpitations or irregular heartbeat
- Muscle weakness or numbness
- Fatigue and lethargy
- Nausea or vomiting

- Difficulty breathing (in extreme cases)

Recognizing these symptoms early and responding with dietary and medical intervention is essential.

The Role of Diet in Potassium Management
A well-managed diet can make a profound difference in regulating potassium levels, especially for individuals with kidney disease or other potassium-sensitive conditions. A low-potassium diet doesn't mean eliminating all fruits, vegetables, or whole grains—it means making strategic food choices, cooking methods (such as leaching vegetables), and portion controls to stay within safe potassium limits.

This cookbook is designed to support those efforts. With practical information and flavorful recipes, readers will learn how to enjoy a nourishing and satisfying diet without risking potassium overload. In the chapters ahead, you'll explore food charts, recipes, meal plans, and tips that turn potassium management into a sustainable and enjoyable lifestyle.

What Is Hyperkalemia?

Hyperkalemia is a medical term that refers to an abnormally high level of potassium in the blood. While potassium is an essential mineral that supports various bodily functions—such as regulating heart rhythm, facilitating nerve signaling, and aiding muscle contraction—too much of it can be dangerous, and in severe cases, even life-threatening. The condition is most commonly associated with impaired kidney function, but it can also be triggered by certain medications, chronic diseases, or dietary imbalances.

Under normal circumstances, the kidneys maintain potassium levels by filtering excess potassium out of the bloodstream and excreting it in the urine. When the kidneys are damaged or compromised, as in chronic kidney disease (CKD), this filtration process is impaired, and potassium begins to accumulate in the body. Hyperkalemia is typically diagnosed when blood potassium levels rise above 5.0 milliequivalents per liter (mEq/L), with levels above 6.0 mEq/L considered potentially dangerous and requiring immediate medical intervention.

Causes of Hyperkalemia
The causes of hyperkalemia are multifactorial and can include both acute and chronic health conditions. Common causes include:

- Chronic Kidney Disease: When the kidneys lose the ability to properly filter waste, potassium levels can quickly build up.

- Medications: Some medications can impair potassium excretion or promote potassium retention. These include:

  1. ACE inhibitors (e.g., lisinopril)
  2. ARBs (e.g., losartan)
  3. Potassium-sparing diuretics (e.g., spironolactone)
  4. NSAIDs (e.g., ibuprofen)

- Adrenal Insufficiency: Conditions like Addison's disease can reduce hormone production that is essential for potassium regulation.

- **Uncontrolled Diabetes:** High blood sugar levels and acidosis can alter the way potassium moves in and out of cells.

- **Excessive Dietary Potassium:** Consuming a large amount of potassium-rich foods or supplements can contribute, particularly in individuals with impaired renal function.

- **Trauma or Severe Injury:** Breakdown of muscle tissue releases intracellular potassium into the bloodstream, a condition known as rhabdomyolysis.

Symptoms of Hyperkalemia

Hyperkalemia can be deceptive, as it may not present with symptoms in its early stages. When symptoms do occur, they can range from mild to severe and often resemble other conditions, making diagnosis more difficult without blood tests.

Common symptoms include:

- Muscle weakness or fatigue
- Numbness or tingling sensations
- Nausea or vomiting
- Irregular heartbeat (arrhythmias)
- Shortness of breath
- Chest pain
- Palpitations or skipped heartbeats

In extreme cases, hyperkalemia can lead to cardiac arrest, which is why managing potassium levels is critical for individuals at risk.

Diagnosing and Monitoring Hyperkalemia

Diagnosis of hyperkalemia is done through a serum potassium blood test, often as part of a comprehensive metabolic panel. When hyperkalemia is suspected or detected, further tests may be ordered to identify the underlying cause. These might include kidney function tests, blood sugar levels, ECG (electrocardiogram), and tests for adrenal function.

For people with chronic conditions, routine monitoring of potassium levels becomes a critical component of long-term health management. In such cases, physicians and dietitians often recommend dietary modifications as a non-pharmacological strategy to keep potassium levels within a safe range.

Dietary Management of Hyperkalemia

One of the most effective and sustainable ways to manage hyperkalemia is through a low-potassium diet. This involves:

- Avoiding high-potassium foods (e.g., bananas, oranges, potatoes, avocados, spinach, tomatoes)
- Choosing lower-potassium alternatives (e.g., apples, berries, rice, cauliflower, cabbage)
- Practicing proper cooking methods like leaching, which helps reduce potassium content in vegetables
- Reading food labels carefully to avoid hidden potassium additives like potassium chloride
- Limiting processed foods that may contain potassium-based preservatives

This cookbook is specifically designed to help readers make those dietary changes easier and more enjoyable. From recipe development to a structured 30-day meal plan, every section is built to guide you in managing hyperkalemia safely while still enjoying nourishing, delicious meals.

Partnering with Your Healthcare Team

Managing hyperkalemia requires a collaborative approach between the patient, healthcare provider, and often a registered dietitian. Medication adjustments, regular lab tests, and individualized dietary advice should all be part of your care plan. Never attempt to self-treat hyperkalemia through diet alone without professional guidance, as both high and low potassium levels can be dangerous.

In the next section, we'll explore "The Importance of a Low-Potassium Diet", including how it supports not only kidney function but overall cardiovascular and muscular health.

The Importance of a Low-Potassium Diet

For individuals diagnosed with chronic kidney disease, adrenal insufficiency, heart conditions, or those taking certain medications, a low-potassium diet is not just a recommendation, it is a lifesaving strategy. While potassium is an essential mineral that plays vital roles in muscle function, nerve transmission, and heart rhythm, an excess of it in the blood, known as hyperkalemia, can pose serious health risks, especially when left unmanaged. Adopting a low-potassium diet is a proactive and effective way to help the body maintain electrolyte balance and reduce the burden on compromised kidneys or systems struggling to regulate potassium efficiently.

Who Needs a Low-Potassium Diet?

A low-potassium diet is commonly prescribed for people in the following categories:

- **Chronic Kidney Disease (CKD):** As kidney function declines, the ability to excrete potassium diminishes. A low-potassium diet becomes essential to prevent dangerous accumulation in the blood.

- **Dialysis Patients:** Individuals on dialysis need to manage their potassium intake carefully between treatments to avoid life-threatening spikes.

- **Heart Failure Patients:** Certain heart medications, such as ACE inhibitors or potassium-sparing diuretics, can increase potassium levels. A controlled diet helps balance this effect.

- **People with Adrenal Disorders:** In conditions like Addison's disease, the adrenal glands fail to produce enough aldosterone, a hormone that helps regulate potassium levels.

Those with Uncontrolled Diabetes: Fluctuations in blood sugar can affect potassium distribution in the body, making dietary regulation necessary.

In each of these cases, dietary intervention becomes a powerful tool for both preventing complications and supporting overall health.

Benefits of a Low-Potassium Diet

- **Prevents Cardiac Complications:** Excess potassium disrupts the electrical signaling in the heart, leading to arrhythmias, palpitations, or in severe cases, cardiac arrest. A low-potassium diet helps maintain safe levels and protects heart health.
- **Supports Kidney Function:** Reducing dietary potassium helps minimize the workload of impaired kidneys. It allows for better fluid balance and decreases the likelihood of potassium toxicity.
- **Improves Muscle and Nerve Function:** Muscle cramps, weakness, and numbness are common symptoms of hyperkalemia. By keeping potassium levels within a healthy range, these discomforts are reduced or avoided.
- **Enhances Quality of Life:** Anxiety around food can be common for those managing chronic illness. A structured low-potassium diet, like the one outlined in this cookbook, empowers individuals to eat with confidence and peace of mind.
- **Reduces Hospitalizations:** Severe hyperkalemia often requires emergency treatment. Consistent potassium management through diet can help reduce the frequency of urgent medical interventions and hospital visits.

Common High-Potassium Foods to Watch For

A wide range of healthy, natural foods are rich in potassium, which makes the diet somewhat counterintuitive at first. Many items that are often labeled as "healthy"—such as bananas, spinach, potatoes, tomatoes, oranges, and avocados are high in potassium and need to be limited or avoided.

Other less obvious sources include:

- Dairy products (especially yogurt and milk)
- Beans and lentils
- Bran-based cereals and whole grains
- Nuts and seeds
- Coconut water
- Chocolate

Many processed and packaged foods also contain potassium additives, such as potassium chloride, used as a salt substitute or preservative. These can significantly raise potassium intake without the consumer realizing it.

Low-Potassium Alternatives

The good news is that there are plenty of nutritious and flavorful alternatives that are lower in potassium. These include:

- Apples, berries, grapes, and peaches (canned or fresh)
- White rice and refined grains (in moderation)
- Cabbage, cauliflower, zucchini, and green beans
- Unsalted butter or non-dairy alternatives
- White bread and pasta (again, in moderation)

This cookbook carefully curates recipes that incorporate these low-potassium ingredients without compromising on taste or satisfaction. Cooking methods like leaching vegetables—a technique where you boil sliced vegetables in water and drain them to reduce their potassium content—are also featured throughout the book to help make traditionally high-potassium foods safer to consume.

Monitoring and Portion Control

Portion control is just as important as food selection. A food that is moderately high in potassium may still be consumed in small portions if it fits within your daily potassium allowance, typically 1,500 to 2,000 mg per day for those on a restricted diet. Working closely with your doctor or registered dietitian is essential to determine your specific dietary needs and safe limits.

Additionally, tracking your meals using a food journal or mobile app can help keep your potassium intake within range. Over time, you'll learn how to balance your meals and make more informed choices when grocery shopping or dining out.

Empowering, Not Restricting

The goal of this cookbook is to shift the perception of a low-potassium diet from one of restriction to one of empowerment. Yes, there are foods to limit or avoid, but there is also an abundance of flavorful, safe, and satisfying foods to enjoy. With the help of this book's recipes, meal plans, and tips, you can look forward to nourishing your body while minimizing health risks.

Eating well on a low-potassium diet isn't just possible—it can be enjoyable, healing, and deeply rewarding.

Identifying High and Low Potassium Foods

Understanding which foods are high or low in potassium is essential for managing a low-potassium diet, especially if you are living with chronic kidney disease, heart failure, or other conditions that increase the risk of hyperkalemia. While potassium is naturally found in many healthy foods, not all potassium-containing items need to be avoided—what matters most is how much potassium is present and how it fits into your daily intake. This section provides clear guidance on identifying high and low potassium foods so you can make informed choices and enjoy your meals without compromising your health.

Why Potassium Content Varies

Potassium is a naturally occurring mineral found in plant and animal cells. Its concentration depends on various factors, including the food's origin, how it's processed, cooked, or stored. Fresh, whole foods generally contain more potassium than their processed counterparts, but additives in packaged foods can sometimes introduce hidden potassium sources that are just as concerning.

When planning meals on a low-potassium diet, it's critical to categorize foods based on their potassium levels. In general:

- High-potassium foods contain more than 200 mg of potassium per serving.

- Moderate-potassium foods contain between 100–200 mg per serving.

- Low-potassium foods contain less than 100 mg per serving.
- This framework helps simplify food selection while preserving a wide variety of options across food groups.

Common High-Potassium Foods (Limit or Avoid)

These foods are naturally rich in potassium and are generally not suitable for those on a potassium-restricted diet unless specifically portioned under a healthcare provider's guidance:

Fruits:

- Bananas (1 medium = ~422 mg)
- Oranges and orange juice
- Avocados
- Cantaloupe and honeydew
- Dried fruits (raisins, apricots, prunes)
- Kiwi and mangoes

Vegetables:

- Potatoes (especially baked or boiled)
- Sweet potatoes and yams
- Tomatoes and tomato-based products (sauce, paste)
- Spinach (cooked = very high)
- Swiss chard and beet greens
- Pumpkin and winter squash
- Artichokes

Legumes & Nuts:

- Lentils, kidney beans, black beans
- Soybeans and tofu
- Peanuts, almonds, and cashews
- Nut butters

Dairy and Animal Products:

- Milk and yogurt (1 cup = ~350-400 mg)
- Cheese (especially processed types)
- Ice cream and pudding
- Fish like salmon and halibut
- Beef liver and organ meats

Other Sources:

- Coconut water (very high)
- Chocolate and cocoa powder
- Bran cereals and whole grains
- Salt substitutes with potassium chloride
- Protein drinks and meal replacements

Common Low-Potassium Foods (Safe Choices)

These foods are generally safe for a low-potassium diet and can form the basis of nutritious and enjoyable meals:

Fruits:

- Apples and applesauce
- Grapes and grape juice
- Berries (blueberries, strawberries, raspberries)
- Pineapple
- Watermelon (in small portions)
- Peaches and pears (especially canned in juice)

Vegetables:

- Green beans and wax beans
- Cabbage (green or red)
- Cauliflower

- Carrots (in moderation)
- Zucchini and yellow squash
- Lettuce, cucumber, and onion
- Eggplant and bell peppers

Grains:

- White rice and pasta
- White bread and refined grain products
- Low-fiber cold cereals (cornflakes, puffed rice)
- Plain crackers and low-sodium snack foods

Proteins:

- Egg whites
- Small portions of lean poultry
- Low-potassium fish like tuna (canned in water)
- Tofu (in limited amounts and leached if needed)

Beverages & Miscellaneous:

- Rice milk (non-enriched)
- Herbal teas
- Lemonade or apple juice
- Unsalted popcorn
- Gelatin and sherbet

Cooking Techniques That Reduce Potassium

In addition to choosing low-potassium ingredients, you can significantly reduce the potassium content of certain vegetables through leaching:

- Peel and cut the vegetable into small pieces.
- Soak them in warm water for at least two hours or overnight, changing the water once or twice.
- Rinse well and boil in a large amount of water.
- Drain the cooking water and do not reuse it.
- Vegetables that benefit most from leaching include potatoes, carrots, beets, and winter squash.

Reading Food Labels for Hidden Potassium

Many packaged and processed foods contain potassium-based additives, which can raise potassium levels significantly without being obvious. Look out for ingredients such as:

- Potassium chloride
- Potassium phosphate
- Potassium lactate
- Potassium citrate
- Monopotassium phosphate

Manufacturers are now required by the FDA to list potassium content on nutrition labels, which makes label-reading easier. As a general rule, foods labeled with less than 100 mg per serving are safe to include.

Personalizing Potassium Intake

Not everyone needs the same level of potassium restriction. Your target potassium intake should be determined by your healthcare provider, typically ranging from 1,500 to 2,500 mg/day. Understanding your personal needs will allow you to incorporate some moderate-potassium foods in appropriate portions while avoiding those that might push you beyond your safe limits.

The recipes and meal plans in this book are all crafted to help you stay within your recommended intake while enjoying a diverse, flavorful diet. With proper planning and smart food choices, you can manage your potassium levels effectively without sacrificing variety or satisfaction in your meals.

Tips for Reading Nutrition Labels

For individuals managing a low-potassium diet, reading nutrition labels is an essential daily skill that empowers better food choices and safeguards your health. Packaged foods—whether frozen, canned, boxed, or bottled—can contain surprising amounts of potassium, sometimes added as preservatives or hidden in unfamiliar ingredient names. Fortunately, with the recent changes in FDA labeling regulations, potassium content is now more consistently included on U.S. Nutrition Facts panels. However, interpreting this information correctly and recognizing hidden sources of potassium still requires care and attention.

This section will equip you with practical tips and strategies to decode nutrition labels confidently and avoid dietary pitfalls that could put you at risk for hyperkalemia or other complications.

1. Locate the Potassium Listing

As of 2020, the U.S. Food and Drug Administration (FDA) requires that potassium be listed on nutrition labels. It typically appears under the line for sodium and is measured in milligrams (mg) per serving.

- A low-potassium food contains less than 100 mg of potassium per serving.
- Moderate-potassium foods range from 100–200 mg per serving.
- Anything above 200 mg per serving is considered high in potassium.
- Always check both the potassium value and the serving size. Many products contain multiple servings per container, which can multiply your potassium intake if you're not careful.

2. Understand Serving Sizes

The potassium content is based on a specific serving size listed at the top of the Nutrition Facts label. Consuming double or triple the serving size will proportionally increase your potassium intake.

Example:
If a soup contains 180 mg of potassium per 1-cup serving and you eat 2 cups, you are consuming 360 mg of potassium—not a low-potassium meal. Portion control is key in managing your total daily intake.

3. Scan the Ingredient List for Potassium Additives

Even if potassium isn't highlighted in the nutrient breakdown, it may be present in the form of additives that don't always affect the potassium number listed, especially in international products or smaller brands.

Look for ingredients such as:

- Potassium chloride (common in salt substitutes)
- Potassium lactate
- Potassium citrate
- Potassium phosphate
- Monopotassium phosphate
- Potassium ascorbate

- Potassium bicarbonate

If any of these appear in the ingredient list, it's a red flag that the item likely contains more potassium than you should consume, especially if it's not quantified on the label.

4. Be Cautious with "Salt-Free" or "Low-Sodium" Claims

Many salt-free or low-sodium products compensate by adding potassium-based salts to enhance flavor. Potassium chloride is commonly used as a sodium replacement and can be dangerous for those on potassium-restricted diets.

Check for the "No Potassium Added" or "Potassium-Free" labels, and always verify with the Nutrition Facts and ingredient list. Products marketed as "heart-healthy" or "sodium-free" can sometimes be surprisingly high in potassium.

5. Check for Daily Value (DV) Percentage

Some labels list potassium as a percentage of the Daily Value (DV), with the DV being 4,700 mg for a healthy adult. However, people with kidney disease or potassium restrictions typically aim for 1,500–2,000 mg per day.

Rule of thumb:

- 5% DV or less = low potassium (safe)
- 10% DV or more = high potassium (limit or avoid)

So, if a product has 470 mg of potassium per serving (10% DV), it's too high for a low-potassium diet unless eaten in very small amounts.

6. Use Smartphone Apps and Databases

When in doubt, use tools like:

- MyNetDiary or MyFitnessPal for potassium tracking
- The USDA FoodData Central for accurate, up-to-date food potassium levels
- Renal-friendly diet apps that categorize foods based on their safety for kidney health

These tools can help confirm values, compare options, and make safer selections, especially when labels are vague or inconsistent.

7. Don't Rely Solely on Claims Like "Healthy" or "Natural"

Many foods labeled as "organic," "all-natural," or "healthy" may still contain high levels of potassium. For instance, organic tomato sauce and natural coconut water are both potassium-rich despite appearing health-conscious.

Always prioritize the nutrient breakdown over marketing claims. "Clean eating" doesn't always mean "low-potassium."

8. Watch Out for Enriched and Fortified Foods

Foods fortified with potassium (often cereals, meal replacements, and protein bars) are often inappropriate for those on a low-potassium diet. Look for warnings like "fortified with electrolytes" or "enhanced with potassium" on packaging.

Chapter 1: Breakfast Delights

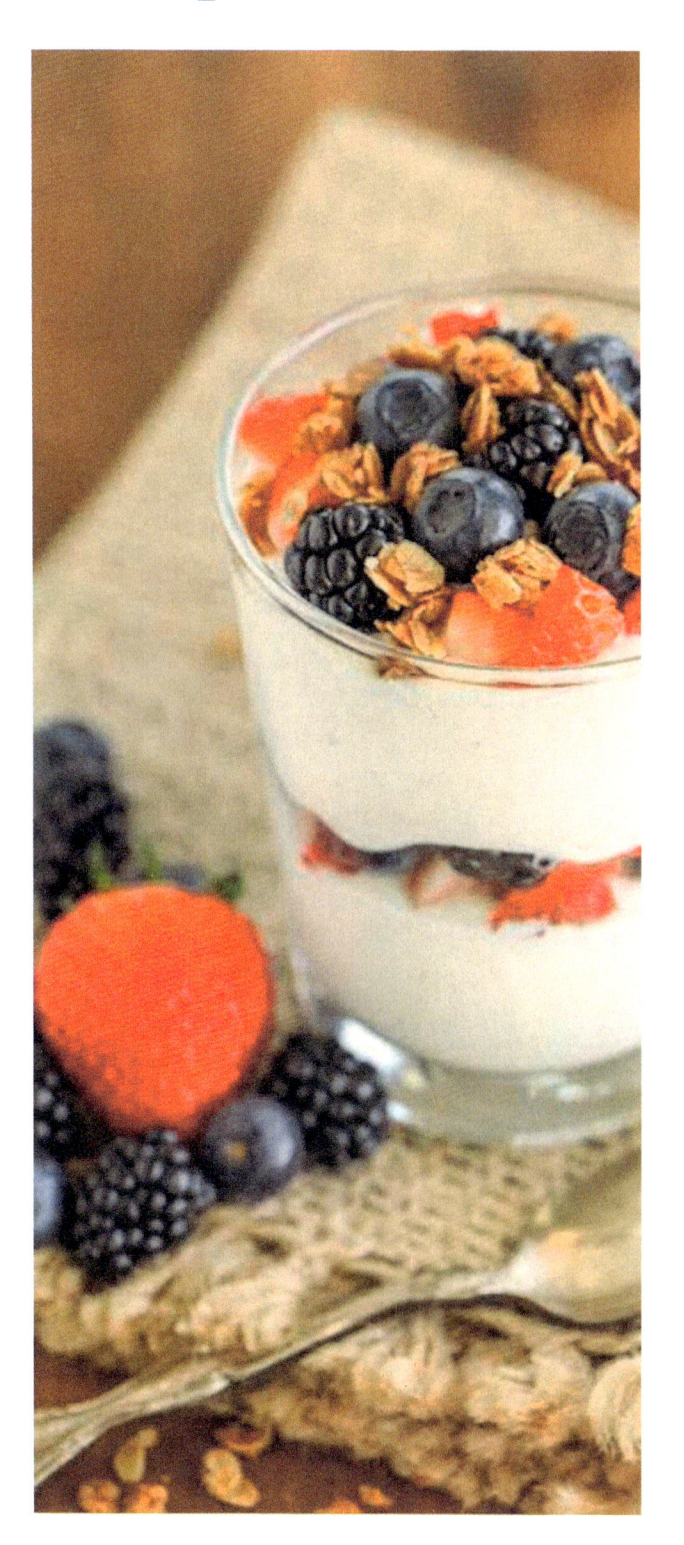

Breakfast is often called the most important meal of the day, and for individuals managing a low-potassium lifestyle, it's also one of the most strategic. A well-balanced morning meal can stabilize blood sugar, energize the body, and set the tone for potassium management throughout the day. While traditional breakfast staples such as bananas, dairy-rich smoothies, and whole-grain cereals might be off-limits or need modification, that doesn't mean your breakfast plate has to be boring, bland, or nutritionally unbalanced.

This chapter, Breakfast Delights, brings a fresh and flavorful approach to low-potassium mornings. Whether you crave something warm and comforting or light and refreshing, this collection of breakfast recipes is designed to support your health goals without sacrificing taste. Each recipe has been carefully created to stay within safe potassium limits while still offering protein, fiber, and essential nutrients needed to start your day strong.

Low-potassium breakfast planning can be a challenge without the right guidance. Many ready-to-eat cereals and high-fiber grain products are unexpectedly high in potassium. Even seemingly harmless fruits like oranges or melons can quickly exceed potassium targets when portion sizes aren't monitored. This chapter removes the guesswork. You'll find easy-to-follow recipes that clearly list potassium content per serving and offer substitutions when necessary.

Herbed Egg White Omelet

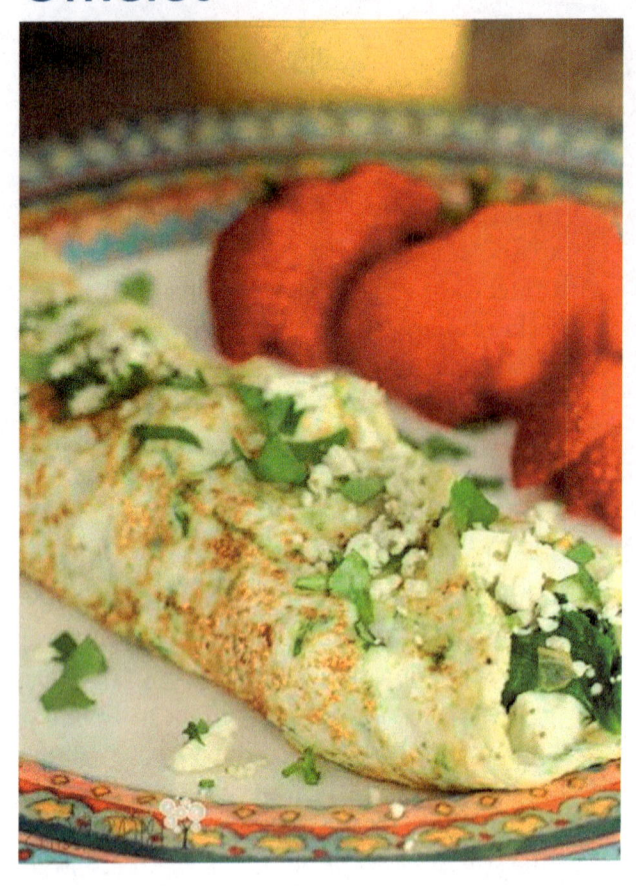

A light yet protein-packed option, the herbed egg white omelet is perfect for a low-potassium breakfast that still delivers on texture and flavor. By using egg whites only and pairing them with kidney-safe herbs and vegetables, this dish becomes a reliable staple for mornings when you want something savory, filling, and easy on your potassium levels. This omelet offers a fluffy consistency, aromatic herbs, and subtle vegetables, creating a wholesome start to your day without overloading your system.

- Preparation Time: 10 minutes
- Cooking Time: 8 minutes
- Serving Size: 1 omelet

Ingredients:

- 4 egg whites
- 2 tbsp chopped fresh parsley
- 1 tbsp chopped fresh chives
- 1 tbsp diced red bell pepper
- 1 tbsp diced zucchini
- 1 tbsp olive oil or avocado oil
- Pinch of black pepper
- Pinch of garlic powder (optional)
- 1 tbsp water (for fluffier omelet)

Instructions:

1. Separate the egg whites from the yolks and place the egg whites in a mixing bowl.
2. Add 1 tablespoon of water and whisk vigorously until frothy.
3. Gently stir in chopped parsley, chives, black pepper, and garlic powder.
4. Heat a non-stick skillet over medium heat and add olive oil.
5. Sauté the red bell pepper and zucchini for 2–3 minutes until softened.
6. Pour the egg white mixture into the skillet over the vegetables.
7. Swirl the pan to spread the mixture evenly.

8. Let it cook for 2–3 minutes until the bottom is set and edges begin to lift.

9. Use a spatula to fold the omelet in half.

10. Cover the pan with a lid for 2 more minutes to ensure it cooks through.

11. Slide onto a plate and serve hot.

Nutritional Values (Approximate):
- Calories: 120
- Protein: 14g
- Carbohydrates: 2g
- Fat: 7g
- Potassium: 110mg
- Sodium: 85mg
- Fiber: 0.5g

Cooking Tips:

- Use a silicone spatula for a gentle flip to avoid breaking the omelet.

- Fresh herbs provide a brighter flavor than dried; if substituting with dried, reduce the quantity by half.

- Adding water to the egg whites helps create a fluffier texture without adding potassium.

Health Benefits:

- Egg whites offer high-quality protein without the potassium found in yolks.

- Parsley and chives provide antioxidants and anti-inflammatory properties.

- A low-fat, low-potassium breakfast that supports heart and kidney health.

Blueberry Pancakes with Maple Syrup

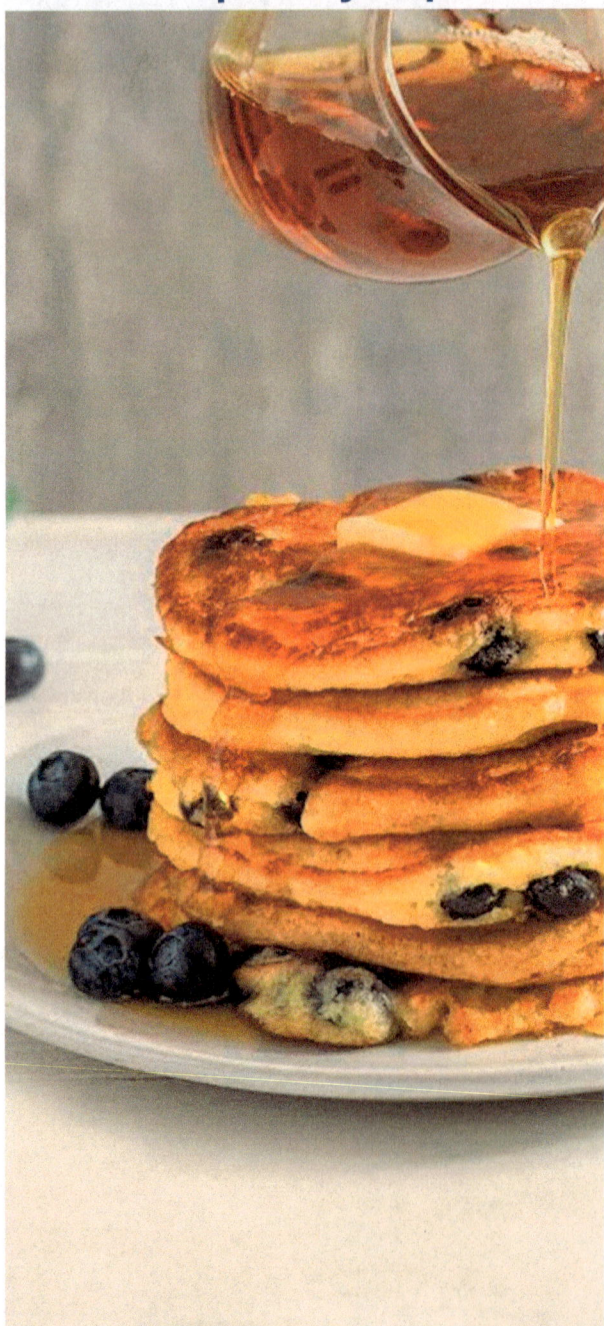

Blueberry pancakes are a breakfast classic—but this low-potassium version ensures you can enjoy them safely without sacrificing flavor. By using all-purpose flour, egg whites, rice milk, and fresh or frozen blueberries in moderation, the potassium content remains low while still delivering a warm, fluffy, sweet breakfast treat. Maple syrup adds a natural touch of sweetness without contributing significant potassium.

- Preparation Time: 10 minutes
- Cooking Time: 12 minutes
- Serving Size: 3 pancakes

Ingredients:

- 1 cup all-purpose flour
- 1 tbsp sugar
- 1 ½ tsp baking powder
- ¼ tsp salt
- 1 egg white
- ¾ cup unsweetened rice milk
- 1 tbsp canola oil
- ½ tsp vanilla extract
- ⅓ cup fresh or frozen blueberries (not wild)
- Maple syrup for drizzling (1 tbsp per serving)

Instructions:

1. In a large mixing bowl, whisk together flour, sugar, baking powder, and salt.
2. In a separate bowl, mix the egg white, rice milk, oil, and vanilla extract.
3. Combine wet and dry ingredients until just blended; do not overmix.

4. Gently fold in the blueberries.

5. Heat a non-stick skillet or griddle over medium heat and lightly grease it.

6. Pour ¼ cup batter per pancake onto the hot surface.

7. Cook until bubbles form on the surface and edges start to dry, about 2–3 minutes.

8. Flip and cook for another 2–3 minutes until golden brown and cooked through.

9. Remove and keep warm; repeat with remaining batter.

10. Serve with 1 tbsp of pure maple syrup.

Nutritional Values (Approximate):
- Calories: 180
- Protein: 4g
- Carbohydrates: 30g
- Fat: 5g
- Potassium: 95mg
- Sodium: 140mg
- Fiber: 1.5g

Cooking Tips:

- Avoid wild blueberries, which have higher potassium levels.

- Use a non-stick pan to reduce the need for added fat.

- For extra fluffiness, let the batter sit for 5 minutes before cooking.

Health Benefits:

- Blueberries are low in potassium and high in antioxidants, supporting cognitive and immune health.

- Rice milk is potassium-friendly and lactose-free.

- Whole-grain alternatives can be used if potassium content is still manageable.

Creamy Rice Porridge with Apples

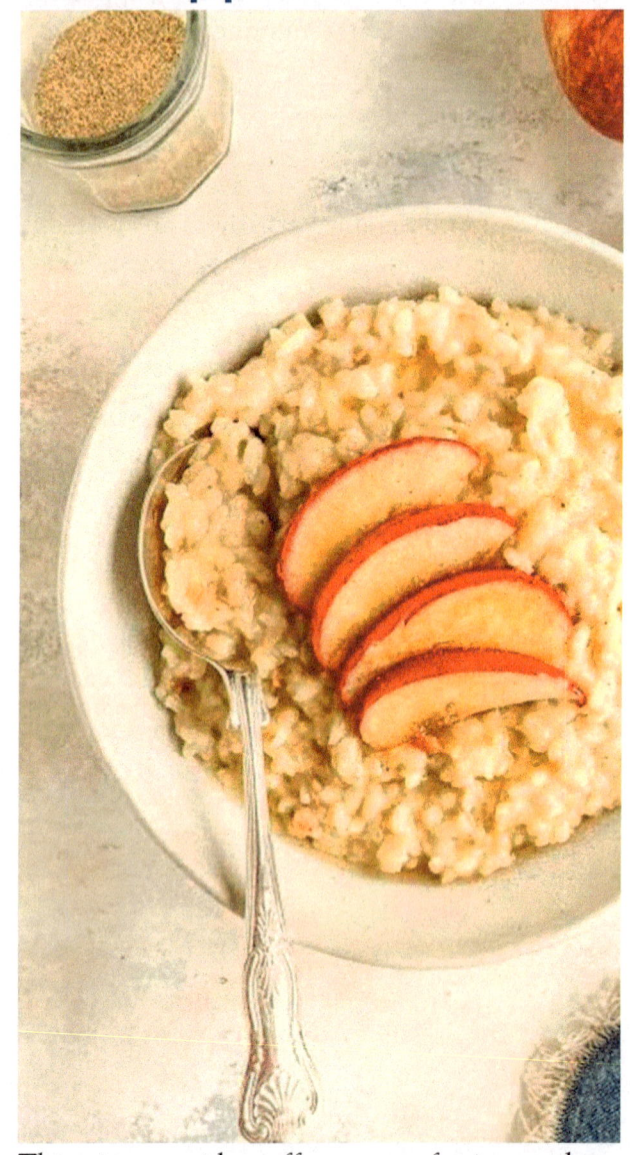

- Preparation Time: 10 minutes
- Cooking Time: 25 minutes
- Serving Size: 1 cup (makes 2 servings)

Ingredients:

- ½ cup white rice (uncooked)
- 2 cups unsweetened rice milk
- ½ small apple, peeled and finely chopped
- 1 tsp maple syrup or agave syrup
- ¼ tsp cinnamon
- ¼ tsp vanilla extract (optional)
- Pinch of salt
- 1 tsp sugar (optional for sweetness)

Instructions:

1. Rinse the white rice thoroughly under cold water to remove excess starch.
2. In a medium saucepan, combine rice and rice milk over medium heat.
3. Bring to a gentle boil, stirring occasionally to prevent sticking.
4. Reduce heat to low and cover partially. Simmer for 20 minutes, stirring occasionally.
5. Add chopped apple, cinnamon, maple syrup, vanilla extract, and salt.
6. Continue to cook uncovered, stirring frequently, for another 5–7 minutes

This rice porridge offers a comforting and creamy texture, ideal for cool mornings or gentle starts. Using white rice ensures low potassium content, while apples add sweetness and fiber without elevating potassium too much. Made with unsweetened rice milk and flavored with cinnamon, this dish is both soothing and nourishing—especially suitable for those managing kidney conditions, gastrointestinal sensitivities, or simply looking for a warm, easy-to-digest breakfast.

until the porridge is creamy and apples are tender.

7. Add a splash more rice milk if a thinner consistency is desired.

8. Serve warm, optionally topped with a sprinkle of cinnamon or apple slices.

Nutritional Values (Approximate):
- Calories: 160
- Protein: 3g
- Carbohydrates: 30g
- Fat: 2g
- Potassium: 90mg
- Sodium: 60mg
- Fiber: 1.2g

Cooking Tips:

- Stir frequently to avoid rice sticking to the pan or forming lumps.

- Use peeled apples to reduce potassium further.

- Add a tiny pat of unsalted butter for richness if your dietary plan allows.

Health Benefits:

- White rice is low in potassium and easy to digest, making it perfect for sensitive systems.

- Apples contribute dietary fiber and pectin, which support gut health.

- Cinnamon may aid in regulating blood sugar, which benefits kidney health over time.

Low-Potassium Smoothie Bowl

- Preparation Time: 10 minutes
- Cooking Time: 0 minutes (no cooking required)
- Serving Size: 1 bowl

Ingredients:

- ½ cup fresh strawberries
- ½ small pear, peeled and chopped
- ½ cup unsweetened coconut milk
- 2 tbsp plain Greek yogurt (low potassium brand or substitute with lactose-free yogurt)
- 1 tsp honey or agave syrup
- 1 tbsp chia seeds (optional)
- 1 tbsp unsweetened shredded coconut (for topping)
- A few fresh mint leaves (for garnish)

Instructions:

1. Place strawberries, pear, coconut milk, Greek yogurt, and honey into a blender.
2. Blend on high speed until smooth and creamy.
3. If the mixture is too thick, add a splash more coconut milk and blend again.
4. Pour the smoothie into a bowl.
5. Sprinkle chia seeds evenly over the top for added fiber and texture.

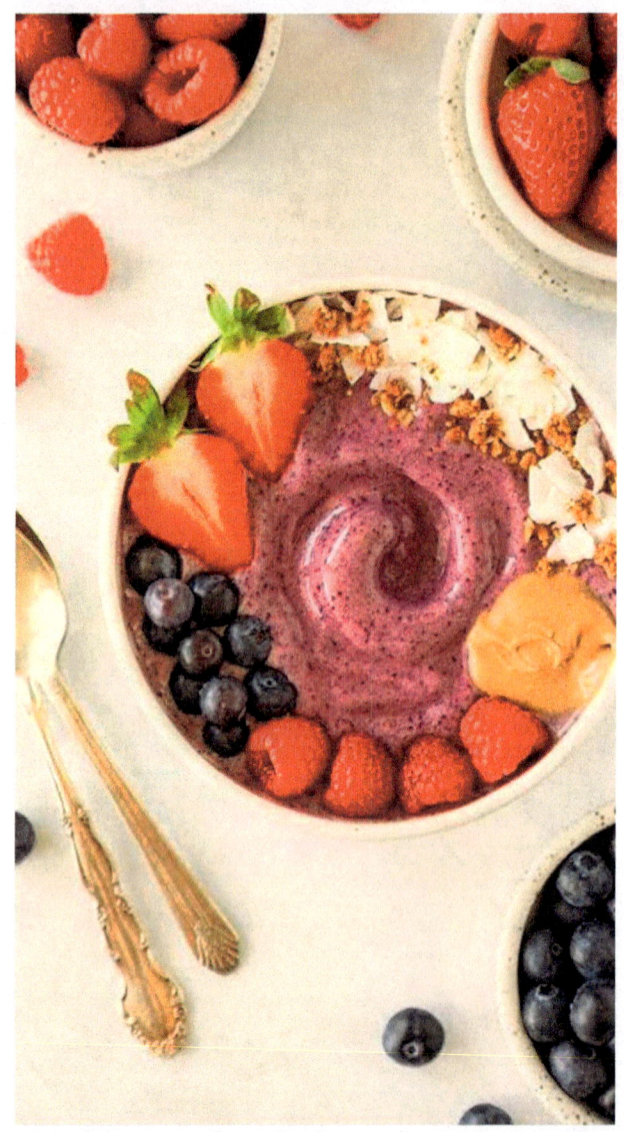

A vibrant and refreshing low-potassium smoothie bowl offers a nutrient-dense and satisfying breakfast option that can be customized easily. By using kidney-friendly fruits like strawberries and pears, along with creamy coconut milk and a touch of honey, this smoothie bowl provides hydration, antioxidants, and energy without exceeding potassium limits. Its colorful presentation makes it visually appealing while delivering fiber and vitamins in every spoonful.

6. Garnish with shredded coconut and mint leaves.

7. Serve immediately for best freshness.

Nutritional Values (Approximate):
- Calories: 170
- Protein: 5g
- Carbohydrates: 25g
- Fat: 5g
- Potassium: 110mg
- Sodium: 40mg
- Fiber: 6g

Cooking Tips:

- Use fresh or frozen strawberries but avoid larger portions to keep potassium low.

- Chia seeds help thicken the smoothie and boost fiber content, but use sparingly.

- Coconut milk provides creaminess without adding much potassium; avoid coconut water which is high in potassium.

Health Benefits:

- Berries and pears offer antioxidants and vitamins critical for immune support.

- Greek yogurt adds protein and probiotics, supporting digestion and muscle health.

- Chia seeds are rich in omega-3 fatty acids and fiber, aiding heart and gut health.

Oatmeal with Cinnamon and Pears

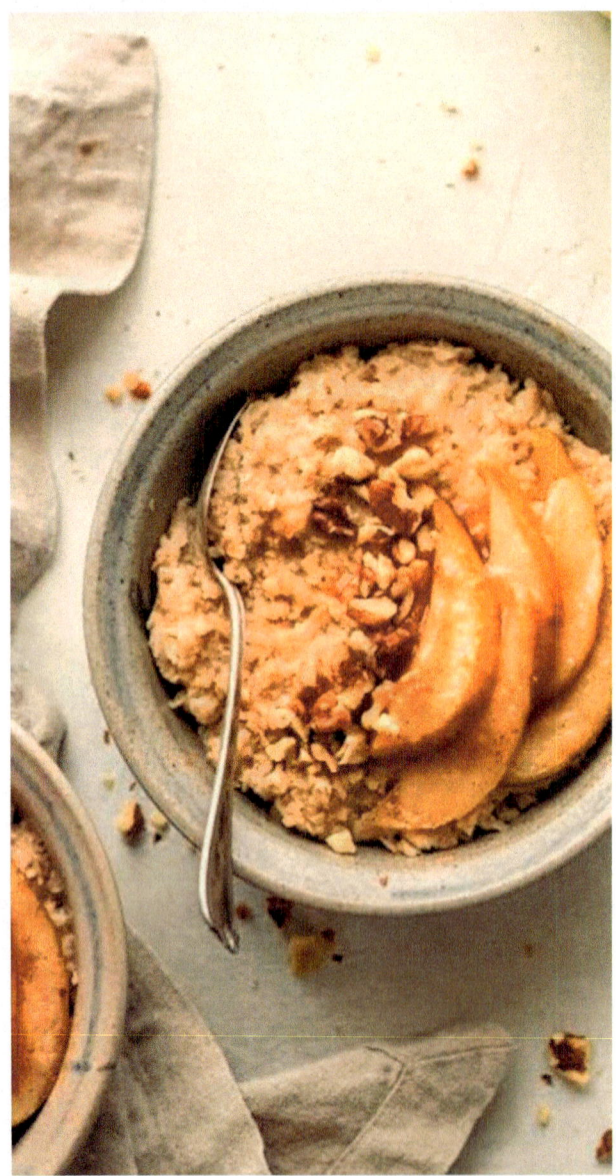

- Preparation Time: 5 minutes
- Cooking Time: 10 minutes
- Serving Size: 1 bowl

Ingredients:

- ½ cup rolled oats
- 1 cup water or unsweetened rice milk
- ½ small pear, peeled and thinly sliced
- ½ tsp ground cinnamon
- 1 tsp maple syrup or honey
- Pinch of salt

Instructions:

1. In a small saucepan, bring water or rice milk to a boil.
2. Add rolled oats and a pinch of salt.
3. Reduce heat and simmer, stirring occasionally for about 8 minutes until oats are tender.
4. Remove from heat and stir in maple syrup and cinnamon.
5. Transfer oatmeal to a serving bowl.
6. Top with sliced pears.
7. Sprinkle extra cinnamon on top if desired.
8. Serve warm.

This comforting bowl of oatmeal is carefully crafted to fit a low-potassium diet by using rolled oats cooked with water or rice milk and topped with sliced pears and cinnamon. The natural sweetness and warmth from cinnamon create a satisfying breakfast that's rich in fiber, slow-digesting carbohydrates, and antioxidants—all while maintaining safe potassium levels.

Nutritional Values (Approximate):

- Calories: 190
- Protein: 5g
- Carbohydrates: 35g
- Fat: 3g
- Potassium: 100mg
- Sodium: 50mg
- Fiber: 4g

Cooking Tips:

- Choose rolled oats over instant oatmeal to avoid added potassium from preservatives.

- Peel pears to further reduce potassium content.

- Adjust sweetness with natural syrups instead of refined sugar for better health benefits.

Health Benefits:

- Oats contain beta-glucan fiber which helps lower cholesterol and supports heart health.

- Cinnamon may improve blood sugar regulation.

- Pears add vitamins and hydration with minimal potassium impact.

Banana-Free Breakfast Muffins

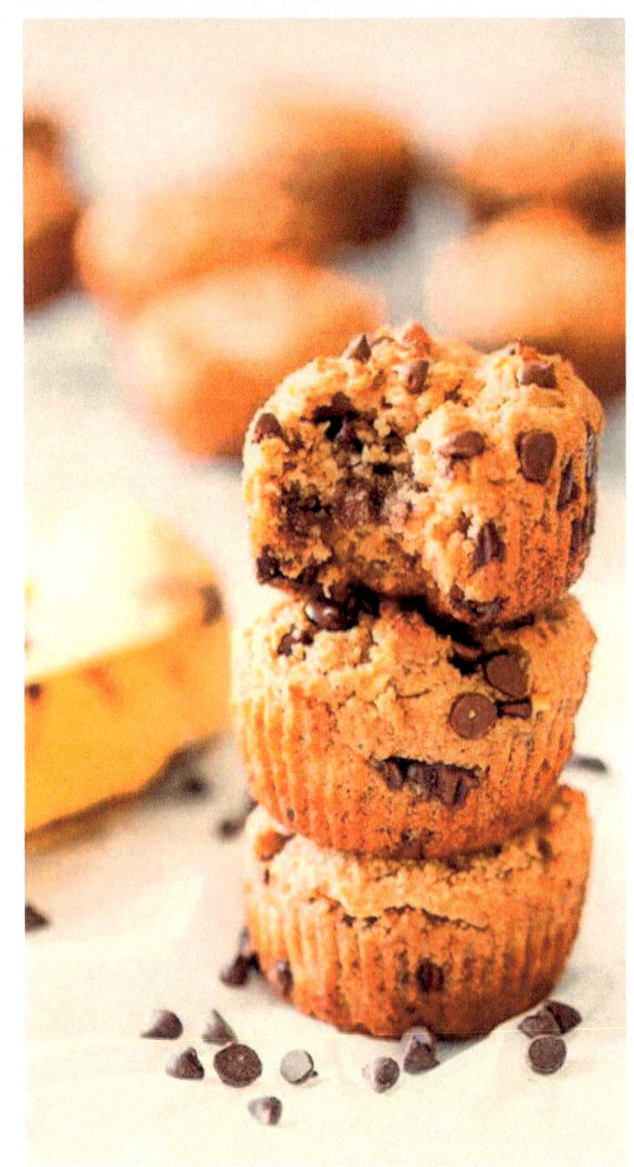

Designed specifically for those who need to avoid high-potassium fruits like bananas, these moist and fluffy breakfast muffins use applesauce and zucchini for moisture and natural sweetness. They're a perfect on-the-go breakfast or snack option, packed with fiber and flavor while maintaining low potassium content.

- Preparation Time: 15 minutes
- Cooking Time: 25 minutes
- Serving Size: 6 muffins

Ingredients:

- 1 ½ cups all-purpose flour
- ½ cup unsweetened applesauce
- ½ cup finely shredded zucchini (squeezed dry)
- ¼ cup sugar or coconut sugar
- 1 tsp baking powder
- ½ tsp baking soda
- ½ tsp ground cinnamon
- ¼ tsp salt
- ½ cup unsweetened rice milk
- 1 tsp vanilla extract
- 2 tbsp olive oil or canola oil

Instructions:

1. Preheat oven to 350°F (175°C).
2. In a large bowl, whisk together flour, sugar, baking powder, baking soda, cinnamon, and salt.
3. In a separate bowl, combine applesauce, shredded zucchini, rice milk, vanilla extract, and oil.
4. Pour wet ingredients into dry ingredients and stir until just combined; do not overmix.

5. Line a muffin tin with paper liners or grease lightly.

6. Divide batter evenly among 6 muffin cups.

7. Bake for 22-25 minutes, or until a toothpick inserted into the center comes out clean.

8. Allow muffins to cool in the pan for 5 minutes before transferring to a wire rack.

9. Serve warm or at room temperature.

Nutritional Values (Approximate, per muffin):
- Calories: 130
- Protein: 2g
- Carbohydrates: 24g
- Fat: 3g
- Potassium: 90mg
- Sodium: 120mg
- Fiber: 2g

Cooking Tips:

- Ensure zucchini is well-drained to prevent soggy muffins.

- Applesauce adds moisture and natural sweetness, reducing the need for added sugar.

- Use fresh ingredients and avoid pre-packaged baking mixes which may contain hidden potassium additives.

Health Benefits:

- Zucchini provides vitamins A and C along with antioxidants.

- Applesauce adds fiber and natural sweetness with low potassium impact.

- These muffins offer a balanced mix of carbs and fats for sustained energy.

Applesauce Pancakes with Agave

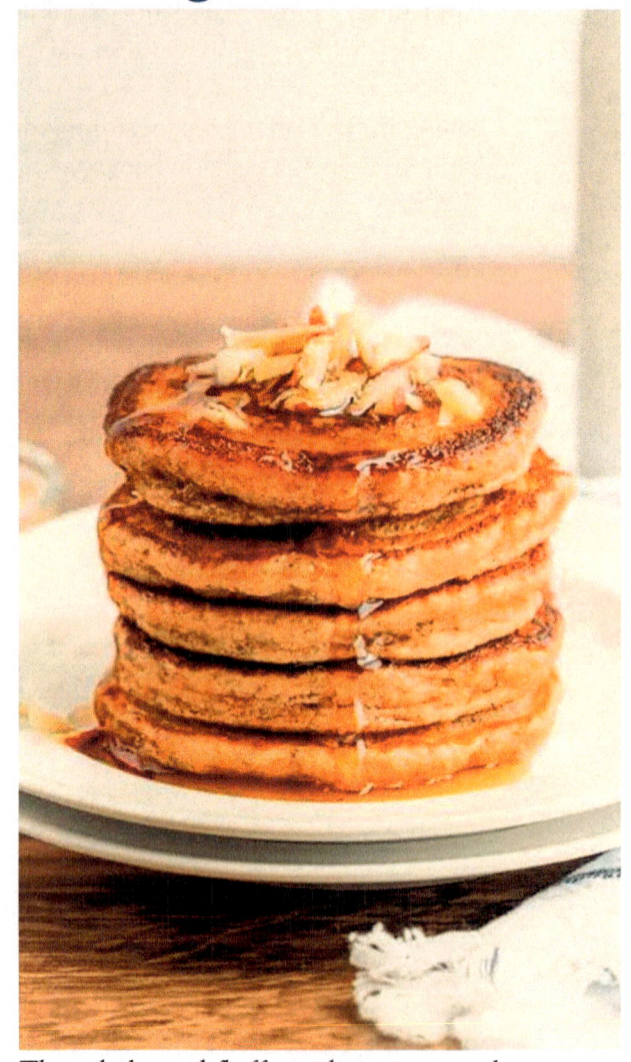

These light and fluffy applesauce pancakes are a delicious low-potassium alternative to traditional banana pancakes. By using unsweetened applesauce, rice milk, and simple pantry ingredients, you get a wholesome breakfast that's both kidney-friendly and crowd-pleasing. Agave syrup adds a mild sweetness without overwhelming the palate or potassium limits.

- Preparation Time: 10 minutes
- Cooking Time: 12 minutes
- Serving Size: 3 pancakes

Ingredients:

- 1 cup all-purpose flour
- 1 tsp baking powder
- ¼ tsp salt
- 1 cup unsweetened applesauce
- ¾ cup unsweetened rice milk
- 1 tbsp olive oil or canola oil
- 1 tsp vanilla extract
- Agave syrup for drizzling (1 tbsp per serving)

Instructions:

1. In a bowl, whisk together flour, baking powder, and salt.
2. In another bowl, combine applesauce, rice milk, oil, and vanilla extract.
3. Gradually add wet ingredients to dry ingredients, mixing until just combined.
4. Heat a non-stick skillet or griddle over medium heat and lightly grease it.
5. Pour ¼ cup batter per pancake onto the skillet.
6. Cook 2–3 minutes until bubbles form on the surface and edges are set.
7. Flip carefully and cook for another 2 minutes until golden brown.

8. Keep pancakes warm while cooking the remaining batter.

9. Serve stacked with agave syrup drizzled on top.

Nutritional Values (Approximate):
- Calories: 170
- Protein: 3g
- Carbohydrates: 35g
- Fat: 4g
- Potassium: 100mg
- Sodium: 130mg
- Fiber: 1.5g

Cooking Tips:

- Do not overmix batter to keep pancakes tender.

- Use unsweetened applesauce to avoid added sugars and excess potassium.

- Serve with fresh low-potassium fruit for added texture and flavor.

Health Benefits:

- Applesauce is a good source of antioxidants and fiber.

- Rice milk provides a lactose-free and low-potassium dairy alternative.

- Pancakes made with simple ingredients support energy levels without excess potassium load.

Low-Potassium Granola Parfait

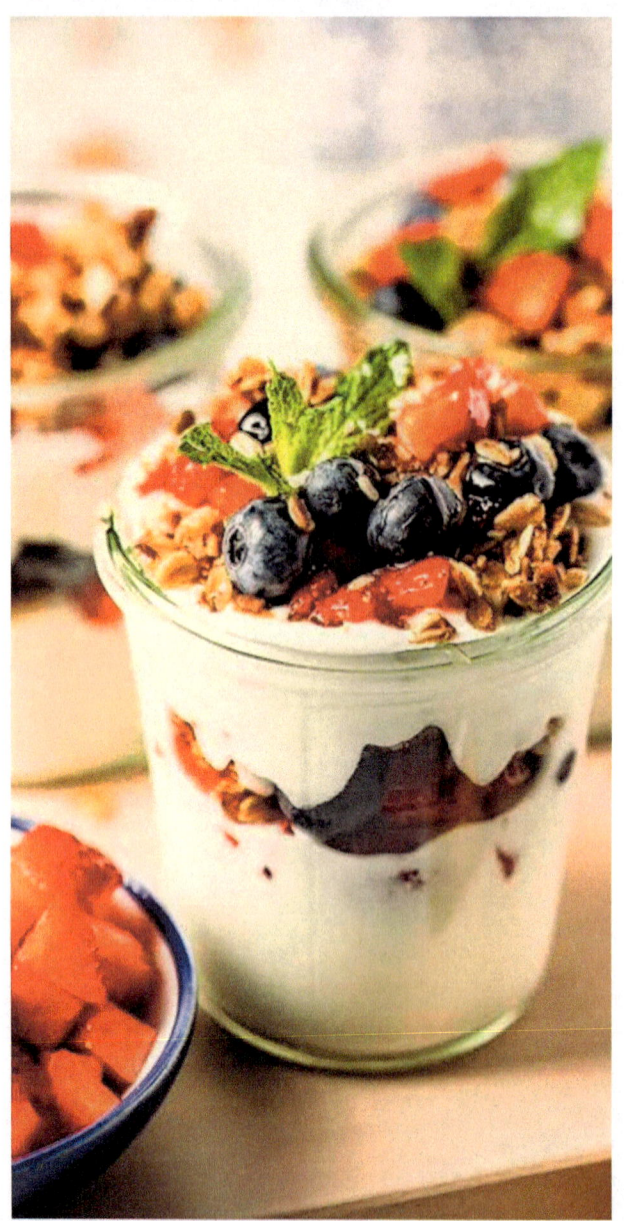

This delightful granola parfait is a layered breakfast treat combining low-potassium granola, creamy lactose-free yogurt, and fresh berries. It offers a crunchy texture balanced with smoothness and natural sweetness. Perfect for those who need to watch potassium intake but still crave a nutritious and satisfying morning meal, this parfait is rich in protein, fiber, and antioxidants, while remaining gentle on the kidneys.

- Preparation Time: 10 minutes
- Cooking Time: 0 minutes (no cooking required)
- Serving Size: 1 parfait

Ingredients:

- ½ cup low-potassium granola (homemade or store-bought without nuts or high-potassium seeds)

- 1 cup lactose-free plain yogurt or Greek yogurt (check potassium content)

- ½ cup fresh blueberries or raspberries

- 1 tsp pure maple syrup or honey (optional)

- A few fresh mint leaves (for garnish)

Instructions:

1. In a clear glass or bowl, spoon ¼ cup yogurt as the first layer.

2. Add a layer of 2 tablespoons of granola on top of the yogurt.

3. Add a layer of fresh berries over the granola.

4. Repeat layering with remaining yogurt, granola, and berries.

5. Drizzle maple syrup or honey on the top layer if desired for extra sweetness.

6. Garnish with fresh mint leaves for color and aroma.

7. Serve immediately to maintain granola crunch.

Nutritional Values (Approximate):

- Calories: 220
- Protein: 10g
- Carbohydrates: 30g
- Fat: 5g
- Potassium: 150mg
- Sodium: 60mg
- Fiber: 4g

Cooking Tips:

- Use granola carefully, avoiding nuts and seeds high in potassium like almonds or pumpkin seeds.

- For homemade granola, use oats, cinnamon, a small amount of honey, and safe ingredients like puffed rice.

- Serve immediately to prevent granola from becoming soggy.

Health Benefits:

- Yogurt provides probiotics which support gut health.

- Berries are rich in antioxidants and vitamin C.

- Fiber from granola and berries helps regulate blood sugar and supports digestive health.

Scrambled Tofu with Bell Peppers

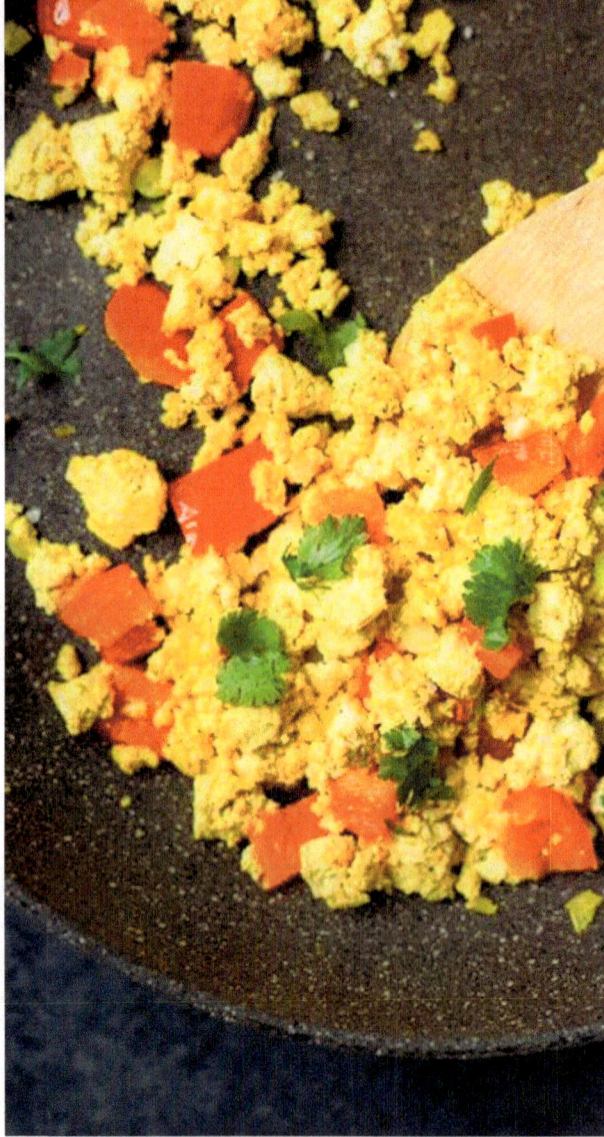

A savory and protein-packed alternative to traditional scrambled eggs, this low-potassium scrambled tofu recipe uses firm tofu and colorful bell peppers to create a flavorful and nutrient-rich breakfast. It's ideal for those avoiding animal proteins or looking for a vegan-friendly option while maintaining low potassium intake.

- Preparation Time: 10 minutes
- Cooking Time: 12 minutes
- Serving Size: 2 servings

Ingredients:

- 1 block (about 14 oz) firm tofu, drained and crumbled
- ½ cup diced red and yellow bell peppers
- 1 tbsp olive oil
- ½ tsp turmeric powder
- ¼ tsp ground black pepper
- 1 tsp dried oregano or Italian seasoning
- 1 tbsp chopped fresh parsley (optional)
- Salt to taste (preferably low sodium)

Instructions:

1. Heat olive oil in a non-stick skillet over medium heat.
2. Add diced bell peppers and sauté for 4-5 minutes until tender.
3. Add crumbled tofu to the skillet and stir well to combine with peppers.
4. Sprinkle turmeric, black pepper, oregano, and salt over tofu mixture.
5. Cook for 5-7 minutes, stirring frequently until tofu is heated through and slightly golden.

6. Remove from heat and garnish with fresh parsley if using.

7. Serve warm, optionally with low-potassium toast or avocado slices.

Nutritional Values (Approximate per serving):
- Calories: 180
- Protein: 16g
- Carbohydrates: 6g
- Fat: 10g
- Potassium: 140mg
- Sodium: 80mg
- Fiber: 2g

Cooking Tips:

- Use firm tofu for the best texture; press out excess water before cooking.

- Turmeric adds color and anti-inflammatory benefits while keeping potassium low.

- Adjust seasoning carefully to avoid excess sodium.

Health Benefits:

- Tofu is an excellent plant-based protein rich in calcium and iron.

- Bell peppers provide vitamin C and antioxidants.

- This dish is heart-healthy and suitable for vegetarian or vegan diets.

Rye Toast with Cream Cheese and Strawberries

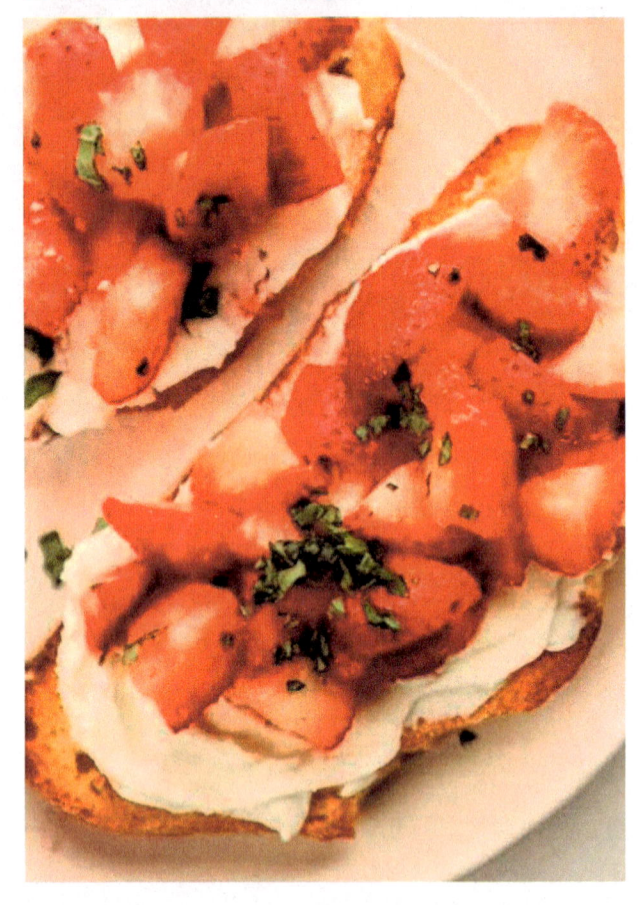

- Preparation Time: 5 minutes
- Cooking Time: 3 minutes (toasting)
- Serving Size: 1 slice

Ingredients:

- 1 slice rye bread (check potassium content)
- 2 tbsp low-potassium cream cheese or lactose-free cream cheese
- 3-4 fresh strawberries, sliced thinly
- 1 tsp honey or agave syrup (optional)
- Fresh mint leaves (for garnish)

Instructions:

1. Toast the rye bread slice to desired crispness.
2. Spread cream cheese evenly over the warm toast.
3. Arrange sliced strawberries on top of the cream cheese layer.
4. Drizzle honey or agave syrup lightly over strawberries if desired.
5. Garnish with fresh mint leaves for added aroma and color.
6. Serve immediately to enjoy the contrast between creamy and crunchy textures.

Nutritional Values (Approximate):

- Calories: 150
- Protein: 5g
- Carbohydrates: 20g
- Fat: 5g
- Potassium: 100mg
- Sodium: 110mg
- Fiber: 3g

Cooking Tips:

- Choose rye bread with no added potassium chloride or preservatives.
- Use fresh, ripe strawberries for optimal flavor and lower potassium than bananas or other fruits.
- Lightly toasting the bread enhances texture without adding potassium.

Health Benefit:

- Rye bread is high in fiber, aiding digestion and blood sugar regulation.

Chapter 2: Wholesome Lunches

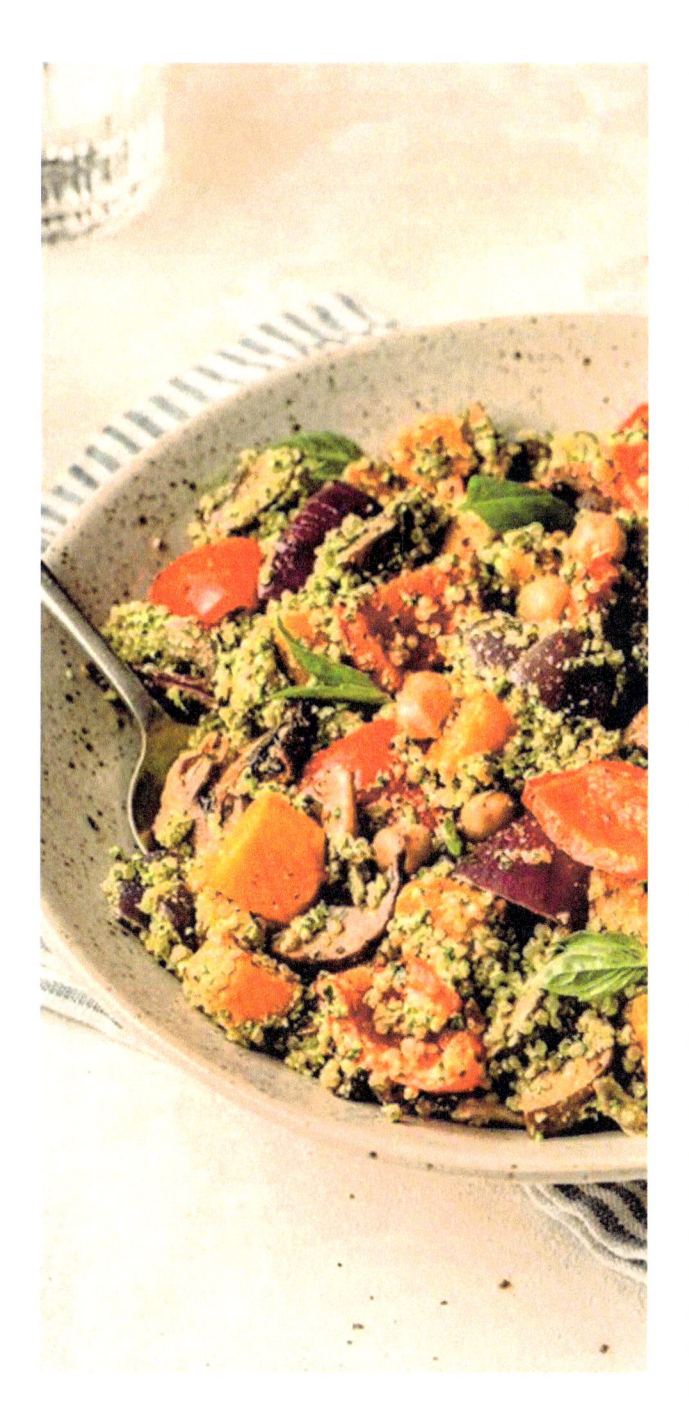

This chapter invites you to explore a variety of delicious, nutrient-packed meals thoughtfully designed to support a balanced low-potassium diet without sacrificing flavor or satisfaction. Lunch is often the day's main meal, and this chapter focuses on wholesome, vibrant dishes that provide sustained energy and essential nutrients while carefully managing potassium levels. From fresh salads and hearty grain bowls to comforting soups and lean protein options, each recipe combines ingredients chosen for their compatibility with a low-potassium lifestyle and their ability to nourish the body.

This chapter emphasizes simplicity and convenience, ideal for busy days, work lunches, or relaxed weekend meals. You'll discover creative ways to prepare familiar favorites with a low-potassium twist, incorporating fresh vegetables, lean proteins, and whole grains that keep you feeling full and balanced. Additionally, practical tips are included to help you customize meals according to your taste preferences and dietary needs while staying within potassium limits.

With attention to both flavor and health, the recipes in Wholesome Lunches offer satisfying combinations that support kidney health, reduce potassium overload, and promote overall wellness. Whether you're new to a low-potassium diet or seeking fresh inspiration, this chapter provides a valuable resource for making lunchtime both enjoyable and nourishing every day.

Grilled Chicken Salad with Cranberries

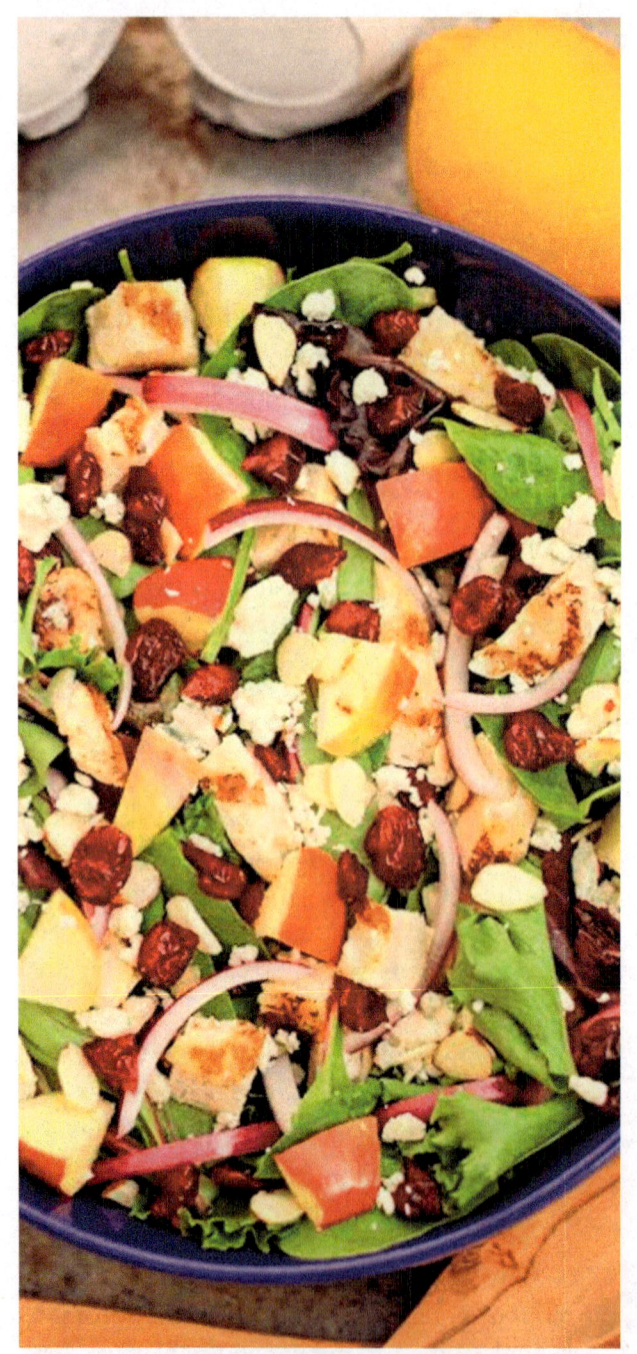

This grilled chicken salad with cranberries offers a perfect balance of lean protein, fresh greens, and a touch of sweetness from dried cranberries. It's a light yet filling meal ideal for a low-potassium diet, combining nutrient-rich ingredients that support kidney health without compromising taste. The salad provides vitamins, antioxidants, and a satisfying texture contrast that makes lunchtime both nourishing and enjoyable.

- Preparation Time: 15 minutes
- Cooking Time: 15 minutes
- Serving Size: 2 servings

Ingredients:

- 2 boneless, skinless chicken breasts (about 6 oz each)
- 4 cups mixed salad greens (lettuce, arugula, spinach - low potassium varieties)
- ¼ cup dried cranberries (unsweetened if possible)
- ½ cup thinly sliced cucumber
- ¼ cup shredded carrots
- 2 tbsp olive oil
- 1 tbsp lemon juice
- 1 tsp honey or maple syrup
- Salt and pepper to taste (use low sodium salt if preferred)
- Fresh parsley or basil for garnish

Instructions:

1. Preheat grill or grill pan over medium-high heat.

2. Brush chicken breasts with 1 tablespoon olive oil and season with salt and pepper.

3. Grill chicken for about 6-7 minutes per side or until fully cooked and internal temperature reaches 165°F (74°C).

4. Remove chicken from grill and let rest for 5 minutes before slicing thinly.

5. In a large salad bowl, combine salad greens, cucumber slices, shredded carrots, and dried cranberries.

6. In a small bowl, whisk together remaining olive oil, lemon juice, honey, salt, and pepper to create a dressing.

7. Drizzle dressing over salad and toss gently to coat evenly.

8. Top salad with sliced grilled chicken breasts.

9. Garnish with fresh parsley or basil leaves before serving.

Nutritional Values (Approximate per serving):

- Calories: 320
- Protein: 35g
- Carbohydrates: 15g
- Fat: 12g
- Potassium: 350mg
- Sodium: 150mg
- Fiber: 4g

Cooking Tips:

- Use fresh cranberries or low-potassium dried cranberries, avoiding those with added sugars or preservatives.

- Let chicken rest after grilling to retain juices and improve tenderness.

- Substitute lemon juice with apple cider vinegar for a different tangy flavor.

Health Benefits:

- Chicken provides high-quality lean protein essential for muscle repair and overall health.

- Cranberries are rich in antioxidants and may help support urinary tract health.

- Salad greens supply fiber, vitamins A and C, and phytonutrients beneficial for immune function.

Turkey and Cucumber Sandwich

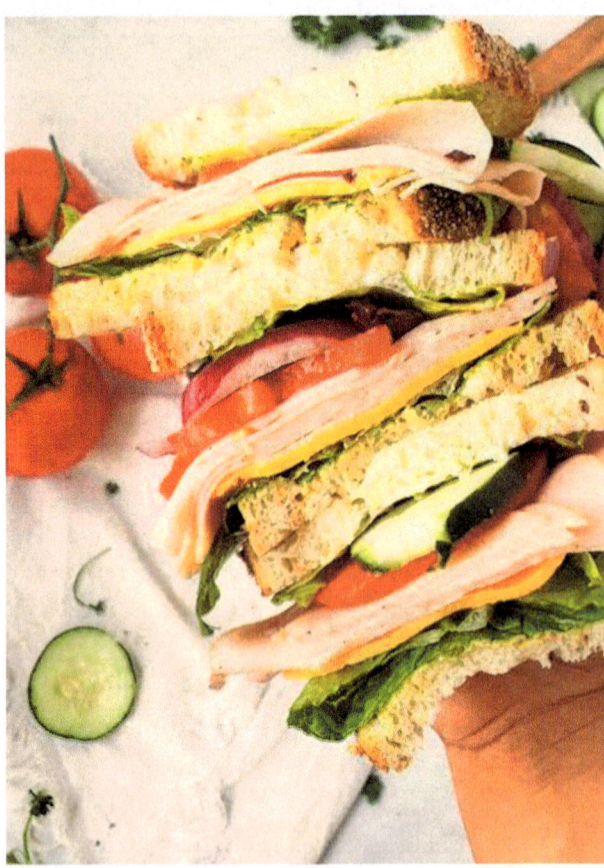

This turkey and cucumber sandwich is a refreshing, protein-rich lunch option that fits perfectly within a low-potassium diet. Featuring lean turkey breast and crisp cucumber slices on low-potassium bread, it's an easy-to-make meal that balances flavors and textures while keeping potassium levels in check. The sandwich is perfect for busy days or packed lunches, offering a satisfying and wholesome meal.

- Preparation Time: 10 minutes
- Cooking Time: 0 minutes
- Serving Size: 1 sandwich

Ingredients:

- 2 slices low-potassium white or rye bread
- 3-4 oz sliced cooked turkey breast (preferably low sodium)
- ¼ cup thinly sliced cucumber
- 1 tbsp low-potassium mayonnaise or lactose-free cream cheese
- 1 tsp Dijon mustard (optional)
- A few fresh lettuce leaves
- Salt and pepper to taste

Instructions:

1. Lay the slices of bread on a clean surface.
2. Spread mayonnaise or cream cheese evenly on one slice of bread.
3. Add a thin layer of Dijon mustard if using.
4. Layer turkey slices evenly over the spread.
5. Arrange cucumber slices on top of turkey.
6. Add fresh lettuce leaves.
7. Season lightly with salt and pepper.
8. Top with the second slice of bread.

9. Cut the sandwich diagonally and serve immediately or wrap for later.

Nutritional Values (Approximate):
- Calories: 280
- Protein: 25g
- Carbohydrates: 28g
- Fat: 7g
- Potassium: 250mg
- Sodium: 300mg
- Fiber: 2g

Cooking Tips:

- Choose fresh turkey breast without added potassium chloride or high-sodium preservatives.

- Peel cucumbers if you want to reduce potassium even further.

- Toast the bread lightly for added texture, but avoid excessive browning which can reduce nutrient content.

Health Benefits:

- Turkey is a lean protein that supports muscle maintenance and repair.

- Cucumbers are hydrating and provide antioxidants with very low potassium content.

- This sandwich is low in saturated fat and a good source of complex carbohydrates.

Quinoa Salad with Roasted Vegetables

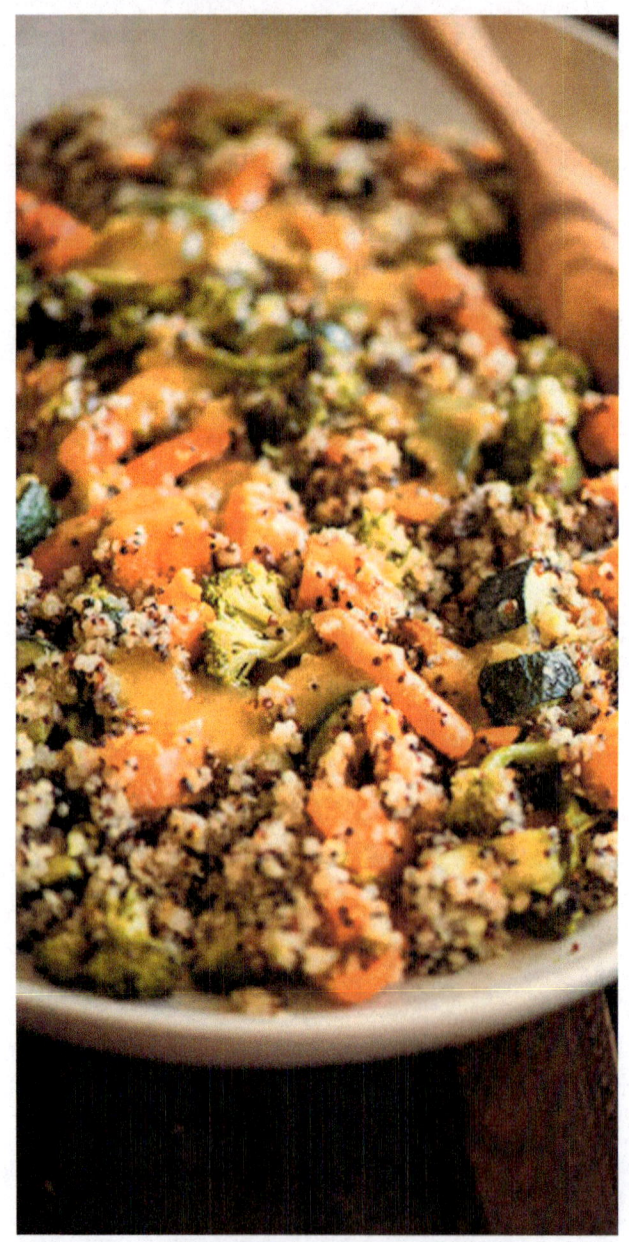

A hearty and colorful quinoa salad loaded with roasted vegetables offers a perfect low-potassium lunch that's both nutrient-dense and satisfying. Quinoa, a complete protein, pairs beautifully with roasted zucchini, carrots, and bell peppers, creating a dish rich in fiber, vitamins, and minerals that support kidney health. This salad is versatile, delicious warm or cold, and ideal for meal prepping.

- Preparation Time: 15 minutes
- Cooking Time: 30 minutes
- Serving Size: 3 servings

Ingredients:

- 1 cup quinoa, rinsed well
- 2 cups water or low-sodium vegetable broth
- 1 medium zucchini, diced
- 2 medium carrots, sliced
- 1 red bell pepper, diced
- 2 tbsp olive oil
- 1 tsp dried thyme or oregano
- Salt and pepper to taste
- 1 tbsp lemon juice
- Fresh parsley for garnish

Instructions:

1. Preheat oven to 400°F (200°C).
2. In a medium saucepan, bring water or broth to a boil. Add rinsed quinoa, reduce heat to low, cover, and simmer for 15 minutes or until water is absorbed and quinoa is fluffy.
3. Meanwhile, place diced zucchini, carrots, and bell pepper on a baking sheet. Drizzle with olive oil, sprinkle

thyme, salt, and pepper, and toss to coat evenly.

4. Roast vegetables in the preheated oven for 20-25 minutes until tender and slightly caramelized.

5. Transfer cooked quinoa to a large bowl. Add roasted vegetables and lemon juice.

6. Toss gently to combine all ingredients well.

7. Garnish with fresh parsley before serving.

Nutritional Values (Approximate per serving):
- Calories: 310
- Protein: 9g
- Carbohydrates: 45g
- Fat: 8g
- Potassium: 300mg
- Sodium: 90mg
- Fiber: 6g

Cooking Tips:
- Rinse quinoa thoroughly before cooking to remove natural bitterness.
- Use low-sodium broth to boost flavor without increasing potassium or sodium.
- Roasting vegetables brings out natural sweetness and intensifies flavor.

Health Benefits:
- Quinoa is a gluten-free complete protein rich in fiber and minerals.
- Roasted vegetables supply antioxidants, vitamins A and C, and dietary fiber.
- Olive oil adds heart-healthy monounsaturated fats and anti-inflammatory properties.

Low-Potassium Lentil Soup

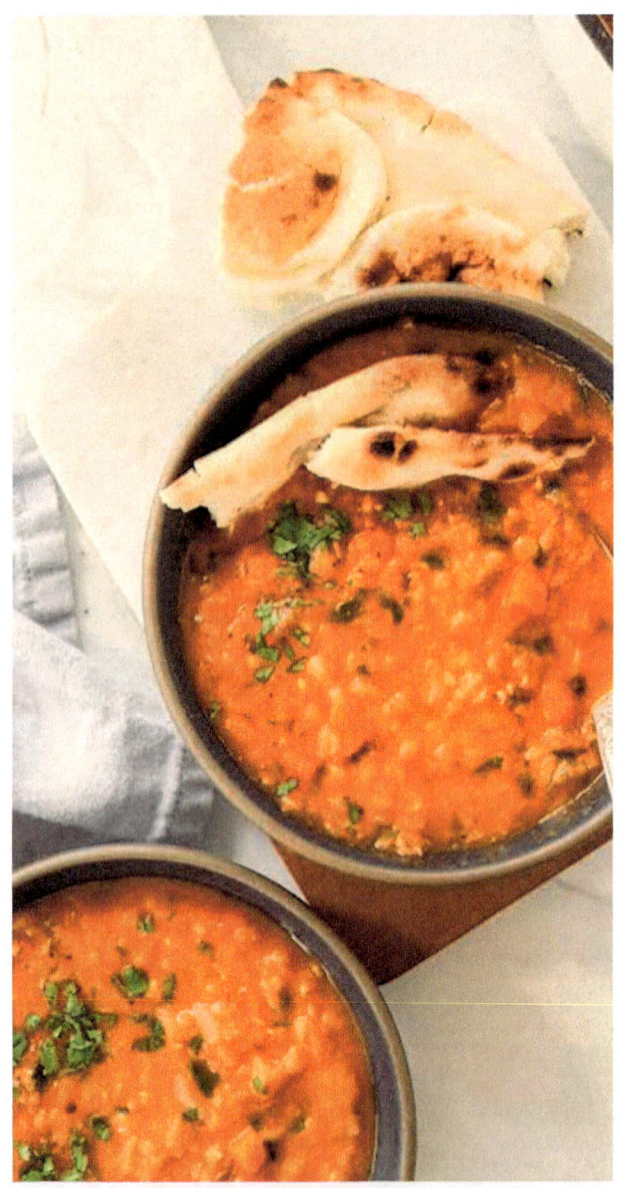

This comforting low-potassium lentil soup is a perfect blend of hearty lentils and aromatic herbs, designed to be gentle on the kidneys while delivering rich flavor and nutrition. Lentils are a great source of plant-based protein and fiber, and this recipe balances the potassium content by using appropriate vegetable choices and careful seasoning, making it ideal for those following a low-potassium diet.

- Preparation Time: 15 minutes
- Cooking Time: 40 minutes
- Serving Size: 4 servings

Ingredients:

- 1 cup brown or green lentils, rinsed
- 1 medium carrot, diced
- 1 celery stalk, diced
- 1 small onion, chopped
- 2 cloves garlic, minced
- 4 cups low-sodium vegetable broth or water
- 1 tbsp olive oil
- 1 tsp dried thyme
- 1 bay leaf
- Salt and pepper to taste
- Fresh parsley for garnish

Instructions:

1. Heat olive oil in a large pot over medium heat.
2. Add chopped onion, carrot, and celery, and sauté for 5–7 minutes until softened.
3. Add minced garlic and cook for 1 minute, stirring frequently.

4. Add rinsed lentils, vegetable broth, thyme, bay leaf, salt, and pepper.

5. Bring to a boil, then reduce heat to low and simmer covered for 30-35 minutes or until lentils are tender.

6. Remove bay leaf before serving.

7. Garnish with fresh parsley and serve warm.

- The vegetable broth keeps sodium low, helping to manage blood pressure.

- This soup supports kidney health by providing nutrients without excess potassium or phosphorus.

Nutritional Values (Approximate per serving):
- Calories: 230
- Protein: 16g
- Carbohydrates: 38g
- Fat: 4g
- Potassium: 400mg
- Sodium: 150mg
- Fiber: 15g

Cooking Tips:

- Rinse lentils thoroughly to remove any debris or dust.

- Avoid adding high-potassium vegetables like tomatoes or potatoes to keep potassium low.

- For creamier soup, partially blend half the lentils and vegetables before combining with the rest.

Health Benefits:

- Lentils provide a rich source of plant protein and fiber to aid digestion and blood sugar control.

Stuffed Bell Peppers with Ground Turkey

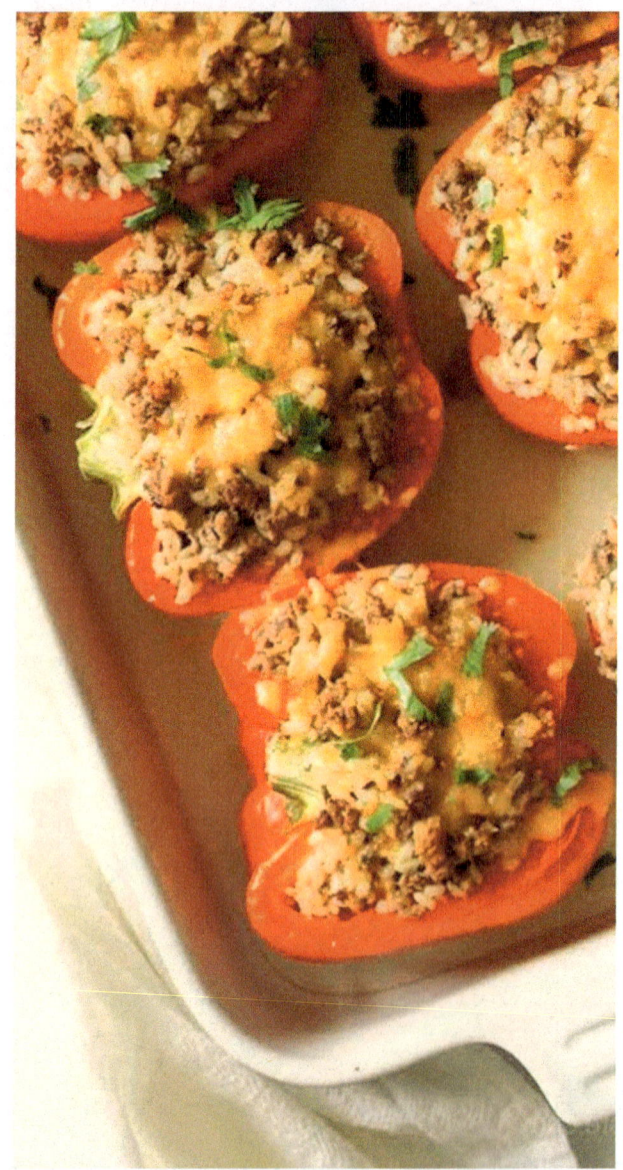

- Preparation Time: 20 minutes
- Cooking Time: 35 minutes
- Serving Size: 4 servings (1 stuffed pepper each)

Ingredients:

- 4 medium bell peppers (red, yellow, or green)
- 1 lb ground turkey (lean, preferably low sodium)
- 1 small onion, finely chopped
- 1 medium zucchini, diced
- ½ cup cooked white rice
- 2 cloves garlic, minced
- 1 tbsp olive oil
- 1 tsp dried oregano
- Salt and pepper to taste
- Fresh parsley for garnish

Instructions:

1. Preheat oven to 375°F (190°C).
2. Cut tops off bell peppers and remove seeds and membranes carefully.
3. In a large skillet, heat olive oil over medium heat.
4. Add onion and garlic, sautéing until fragrant and translucent (about 3-5 minutes).

Stuffed bell peppers filled with flavorful ground turkey and a mix of low-potassium vegetables make a satisfying lunch that's both nutritious and easy to prepare. The bright, tender bell peppers provide a colorful, vitamin-rich base while the turkey offers lean protein, making this dish a balanced option for those mindful of their potassium intake.

5. Add ground turkey, cooking until browned and fully cooked.

6. Stir in diced zucchini, cooked rice, oregano, salt, and pepper, and cook for another 5 minutes.

7. Stuff each bell pepper with the turkey mixture, pressing down lightly to fill well.

8. Place stuffed peppers upright in a baking dish and cover loosely with foil.

9. Bake for 30 minutes or until peppers are tender but still hold shape.

10. Remove foil and bake an additional 5 minutes for a slight browning on top.

11. Garnish with fresh parsley before serving.

Nutritional Values (Approximate per serving):
- Calories: 310
- Protein: 30g
- Carbohydrates: 20g
- Fat: 9g
- Potassium: 380mg
- Sodium: 180mg
- Fiber: 4g

Cooking Tips:
- Choose fresh, firm bell peppers to avoid sogginess.
- Cook rice in low-sodium broth for extra flavor without added potassium.
- For variation, substitute ground turkey with ground chicken or lean beef.

Health Benefits:
- Ground turkey provides lean, high-quality protein essential for muscle repair.
- Bell peppers are low in potassium and high in vitamins A and C, supporting immune health.
- The combination offers a balanced meal with moderate carbohydrates and fats.

Egg Salad Lettuce Wraps

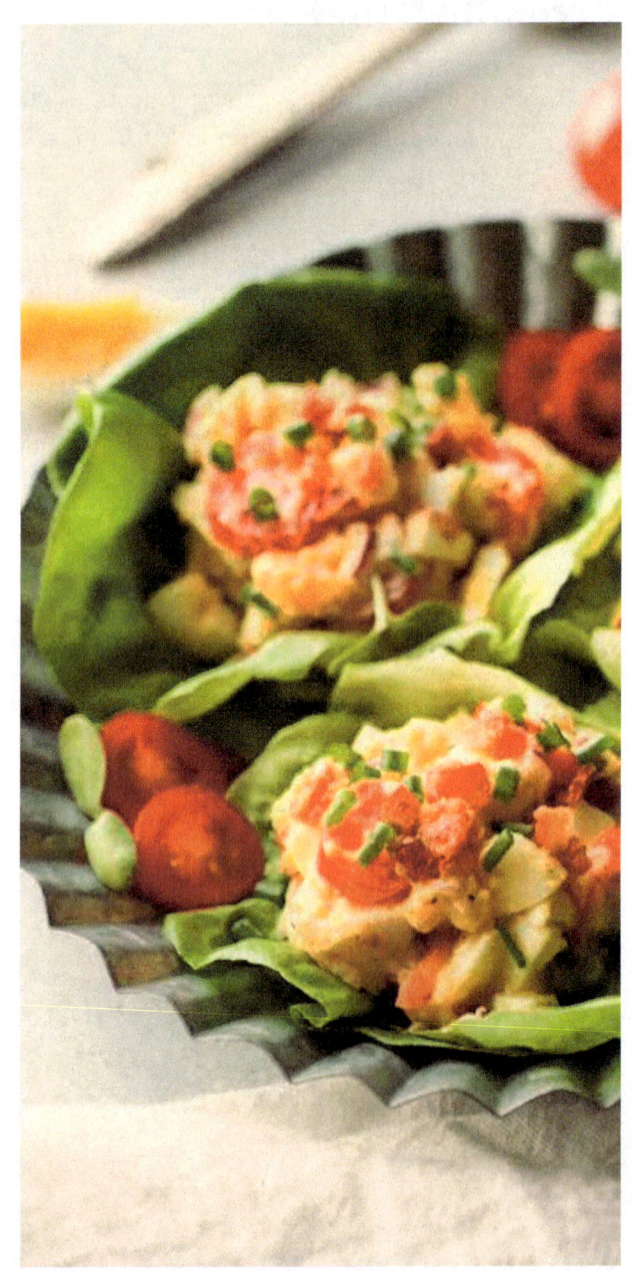

Egg salad lettuce wraps are a light, refreshing lunch option that fits well into a low-potassium diet by replacing high-potassium bread with crisp lettuce leaves. The creamy egg salad made with low-potassium ingredients offers protein and healthy fats, while the lettuce adds crunch and fiber without adding significant potassium.

- Preparation Time: 10 minutes
- Cooking Time: 10 minutes
- Serving Size: 2 servings (3 wraps each)

Ingredients:

- 4 large eggs
- 2 tbsp low-potassium mayonnaise or lactose-free yogurt
- 1 tsp Dijon mustard (optional)
- 1 celery stalk, finely chopped
- 1 tbsp fresh chives or green onions, chopped (use sparingly)
- Salt and pepper to taste
- 6 large butter lettuce leaves or romaine hearts

Instructions:

1. Place eggs in a saucepan and cover with cold water.
2. Bring to a boil over medium heat, then turn off heat and cover pot. Let eggs sit for 10 minutes.
3. Drain and place eggs in cold water to cool. Peel eggs and chop finely.
4. In a bowl, mix chopped eggs with mayonnaise, mustard, celery, chives, salt, and pepper until well combined.
5. Rinse and pat dry lettuce leaves.

6. Spoon egg salad evenly onto each lettuce leaf and fold or roll to form wraps.

7. Serve immediately or refrigerate for up to 2 hours.

Nutritional Values (Approximate per serving):
- Calories: 280
- Protein: 18g
- Carbohydrates: 3g
- Fat: 22g
- Potassium: 250mg
- Sodium: 220mg
- Fiber: 1g

Cooking Tips:

- For creamier egg salad, add an extra tablespoon of mayonnaise or yogurt.

- Use butter lettuce for soft, pliable wraps or romaine for a crunchier texture.

- Avoid adding high-potassium ingredients like tomatoes or avocados.

Health Benefits:

- Eggs are a great source of high-quality protein and essential nutrients such as choline.

- Lettuce adds fiber and hydration with minimal potassium.

- This meal supports muscle maintenance and provides healthy fats for brain function.

Rice Noodle Bowl with Fresh Herbs

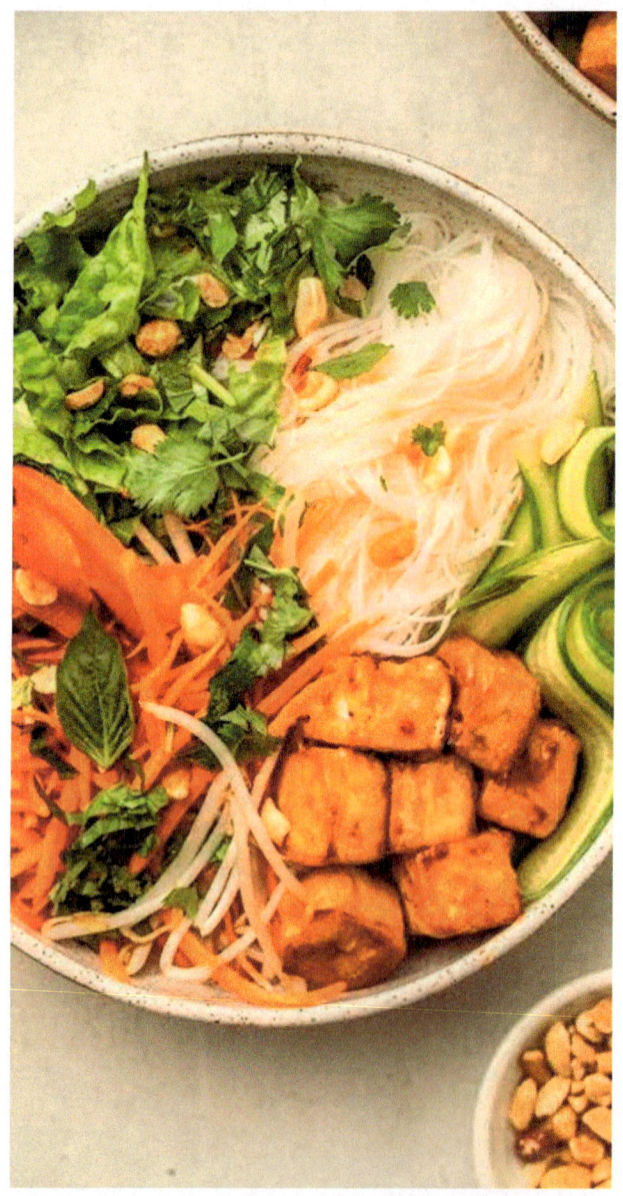

- Preparation Time: 15 minutes
- Cooking Time: 10 minutes
- Serving Size: 2 servings

Ingredients:

- 4 oz rice noodles
- 1 cup shredded cabbage
- ½ cup julienned carrots
- ¼ cup thinly sliced cucumber
- ¼ cup fresh cilantro leaves
- 2 tbsp fresh mint leaves, chopped
- 2 tbsp lime juice
- 1 tbsp low-sodium soy sauce or coconut aminos
- 1 tbsp olive oil
- 1 tsp honey or agave syrup
- Salt and pepper to taste
- Optional: sliced cooked chicken or shrimp (about 3 oz)

This rice noodle bowl is a flavorful, light meal combining tender rice noodles with fresh herbs and crisp vegetables, perfectly suited for a low-potassium diet. The recipe emphasizes fresh ingredients and balanced seasoning to deliver a satisfying lunch that's both nutritious and gentle on potassium levels.

Instructions:

1. Cook rice noodles according to package instructions. Drain and rinse under cold water to stop cooking.

2. In a small bowl, whisk together lime juice, soy sauce, olive oil, honey, salt, and pepper to make dressing.

3. In a large bowl, combine shredded cabbage, carrots, cucumber, cilantro, and mint.

4. Add cooked noodles and dressing to the vegetable mixture and toss well to coat.

5. Add sliced cooked chicken or shrimp if using, and toss gently.

6. Divide into bowls and garnish with extra fresh herbs.

Nutritional Values (Approximate per serving):

- Calories: 290
- Protein: 10g
- Carbohydrates: 45g
- Fat: 6g
- Potassium: 320mg
- Sodium: 200mg
- Fiber: 4g

Cooking Tips:

- Rinse noodles after cooking to prevent clumping and cool the dish.
- Use fresh herbs generously for bright flavor without adding potassium.
- Adjust soy sauce amount to keep sodium low.

Health Benefits:

- Rice noodles are gluten-free and low in potassium, providing energy-rich carbohydrates.
- Fresh herbs and vegetables add antioxidants, fiber, and vitamins.
- Including lean protein supports muscle repair and satiety.

Chicken and Apple Slaw Wrap

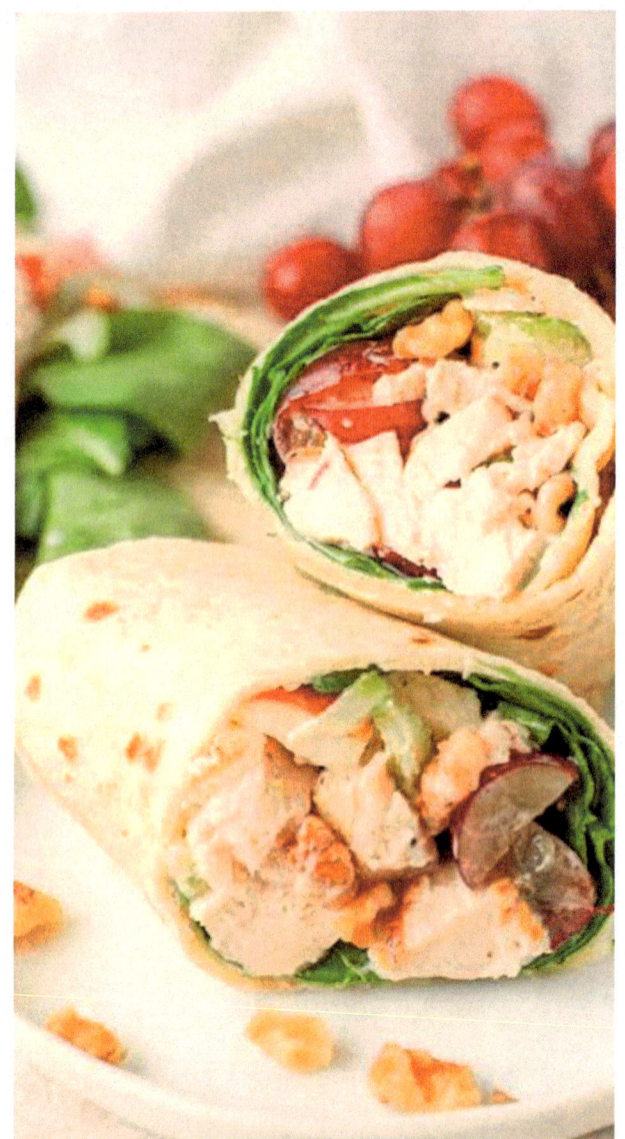

This chicken and apple slaw wrap combines lean protein with crisp, sweet apples and crunchy cabbage, creating a refreshing and nutritious low-potassium lunch option. The blend of textures and flavors makes it satisfying without compromising potassium limits, perfect for a light yet filling meal.

- Preparation Time: 15 minutes
- Cooking Time: 10 minutes (for cooked chicken)
- Serving Size: 2 wraps

Ingredients:

- 1 cooked chicken breast, shredded or diced (about 6 oz)
- 1 cup shredded green cabbage
- 1 small apple, peeled and julienned (low-potassium variety like Fuji or Gala)
- 2 tbsp mayonnaise or lactose-free yogurt
- 1 tsp lemon juice
- Salt and pepper to taste
- 2 large low-potassium tortillas or lettuce leaves for wraps

Instructions:

1. In a bowl, combine shredded chicken, cabbage, and julienned apple.
2. Add mayonnaise and lemon juice, mixing well to coat all ingredients evenly.
3. Season with salt and pepper to taste.
4. Lay out tortillas or lettuce leaves and divide the chicken slaw mixture evenly between them.
5. Wrap tightly and serve immediately or refrigerate for up to 2 hours for chilled wraps.

Nutritional Values (Approximate per serving):

- Calories: 320
- Protein: 35g
- Carbohydrates: 20g
- Fat: 8g
- Potassium: 350mg
- Sodium: 220mg
- Fiber: 4g

Cooking Tips:

- Use leftover cooked chicken or rotisserie chicken for convenience.

- Peel apples to reduce potassium content.

- For a crunchy alternative, substitute cabbage with iceberg lettuce.

Health Benefits:

- Chicken provides lean protein essential for tissue repair and maintenance.

- Apples add fiber and antioxidants that promote digestive health.

- This meal supports energy balance while managing potassium intake.

Tuna Salad on White Bread

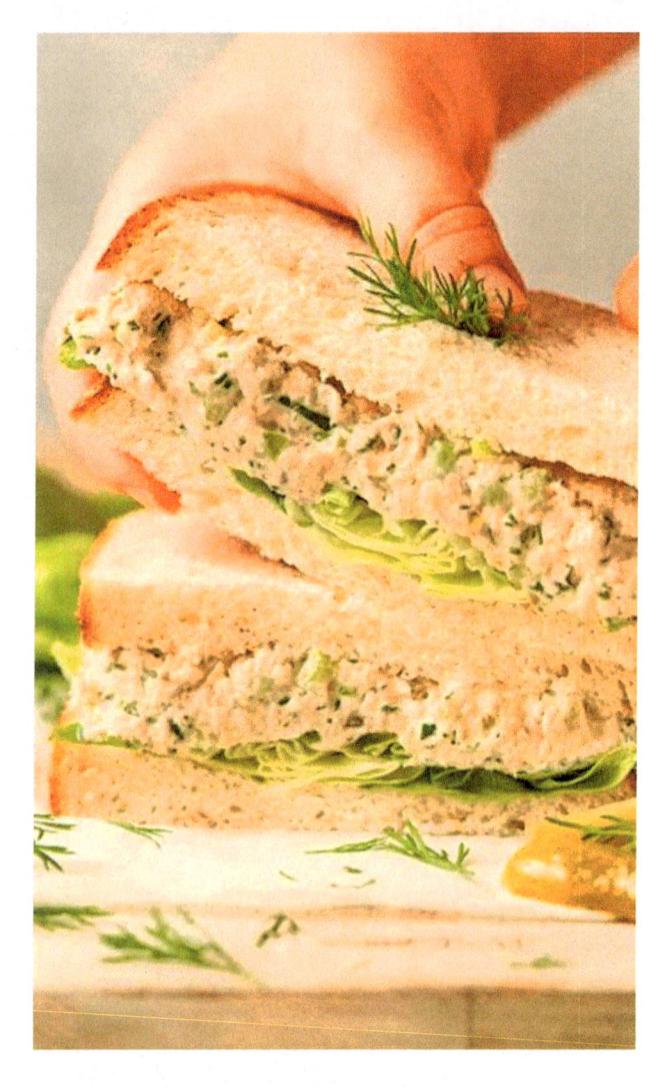

- Preparation Time: 10 minutes
- Cooking Time: None
- Serving Size: 2 sandwiches

Ingredients:

- 1 can (5 oz) tuna packed in water, drained
- 2 tbsp low-potassium mayonnaise or lactose-free yogurt
- 1 tsp lemon juice
- 1 tbsp finely chopped celery
- Salt and pepper to taste
- 4 slices white bread (low potassium choice)
- Optional: lettuce leaves for extra crunch

Instructions:

1. In a bowl, mix tuna with mayonnaise, lemon juice, and celery until well combined.
2. Season with salt and pepper to taste.
3. Toast bread slices lightly if desired.
4. Spread tuna salad evenly over two slices of bread.
5. Top with lettuce if using and cover with remaining bread slices.
6. Cut sandwiches in halves and serve immediately.

Nutritional Values (Approximate per serving):

- Calories: 350
- Protein: 30g
- Carbohydrates: 35g
- Fat: 10g
- Potassium: 300mg
- Sodium: 300mg
- Fiber: 2g

Cooking Tips:

- Drain tuna thoroughly to reduce excess moisture.
- Use white bread as it generally contains less potassium than whole grain varieties.

Couscous Bowl with Zucchini and Carrots

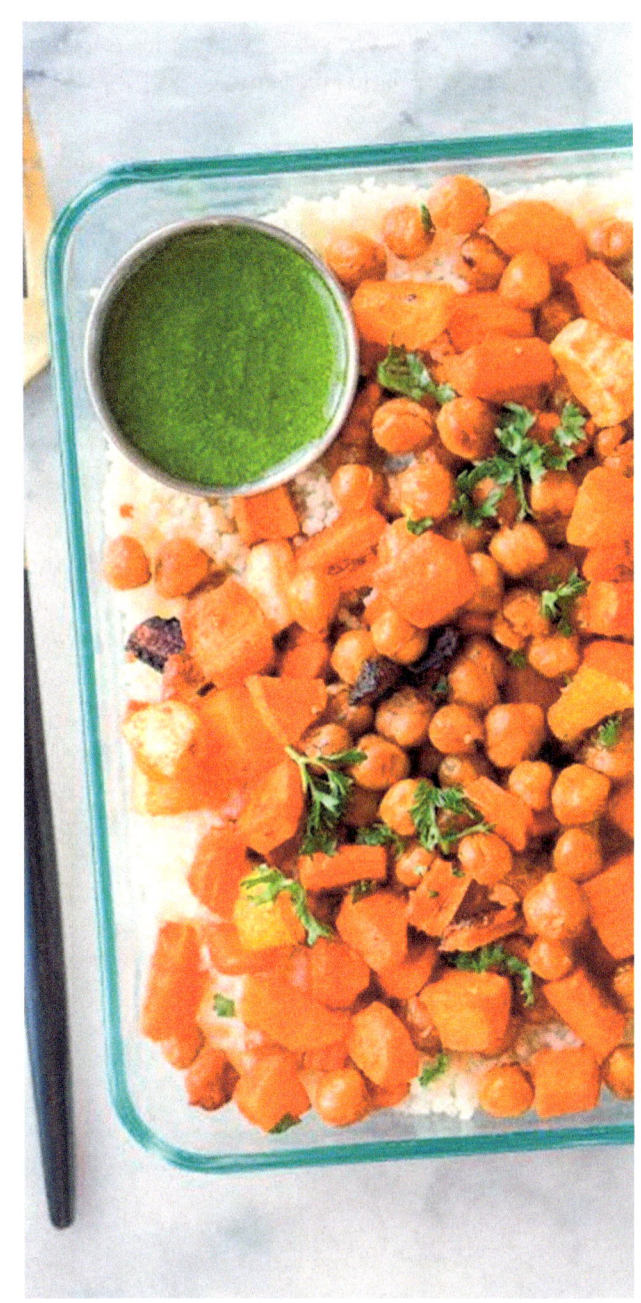

This couscous bowl features fluffy couscous combined with sautéed zucchini and carrots, creating a light and flavorful low-potassium lunch option. The quick-cooking couscous provides carbohydrates for energy, while the vegetables contribute fiber and vitamins without raising potassium levels excessively.

- Preparation Time: 10 minutes
- Cooking Time: 15 minutes
- Serving Size: 2 servings

Ingredients:

- 1 cup couscous
- 1 cup water or low-sodium vegetable broth
- 1 small zucchini, diced
- 1 medium carrot, diced
- 1 tbsp olive oil
- 1 tsp dried basil or Italian seasoning
- Salt and pepper to taste
- Fresh parsley for garnish

Instructions:

1. Bring water or vegetable broth to a boil in a saucepan.
2. Remove from heat and stir in couscous. Cover and let stand for 5 minutes until liquid is absorbed.
3. Fluff couscous with a fork.
4. In a skillet, heat olive oil over medium heat.
5. Add diced zucchini and carrots, sauté for 8–10 minutes until tender but still crisp.

6. Stir in dried basil, salt, and pepper.

7. Combine sautéed vegetables with couscous, mixing well.

8. Garnish with fresh parsley before serving.

Nutritional Values (Approximate per serving):

- Calories: 280
- Protein: 6g
- Carbohydrates: 48g
- Fat: 6g
- Potassium: 300mg
- Sodium: 150mg
- Fiber: 5g

Cooking Tips:

- Use low-sodium broth to enhance flavor without adding sodium.

- Avoid overcooking vegetables to retain texture and nutrients.

- For extra protein, add grilled chicken or tofu.

Health Benefits:

- Couscous provides quick-digesting carbohydrates ideal for sustained energy.

- Zucchini and carrots are low in potassium but rich in antioxidants and fiber.

- This meal supports digestive health and maintains balanced potassium intake.

Chapter 3: Satisfying Dinners

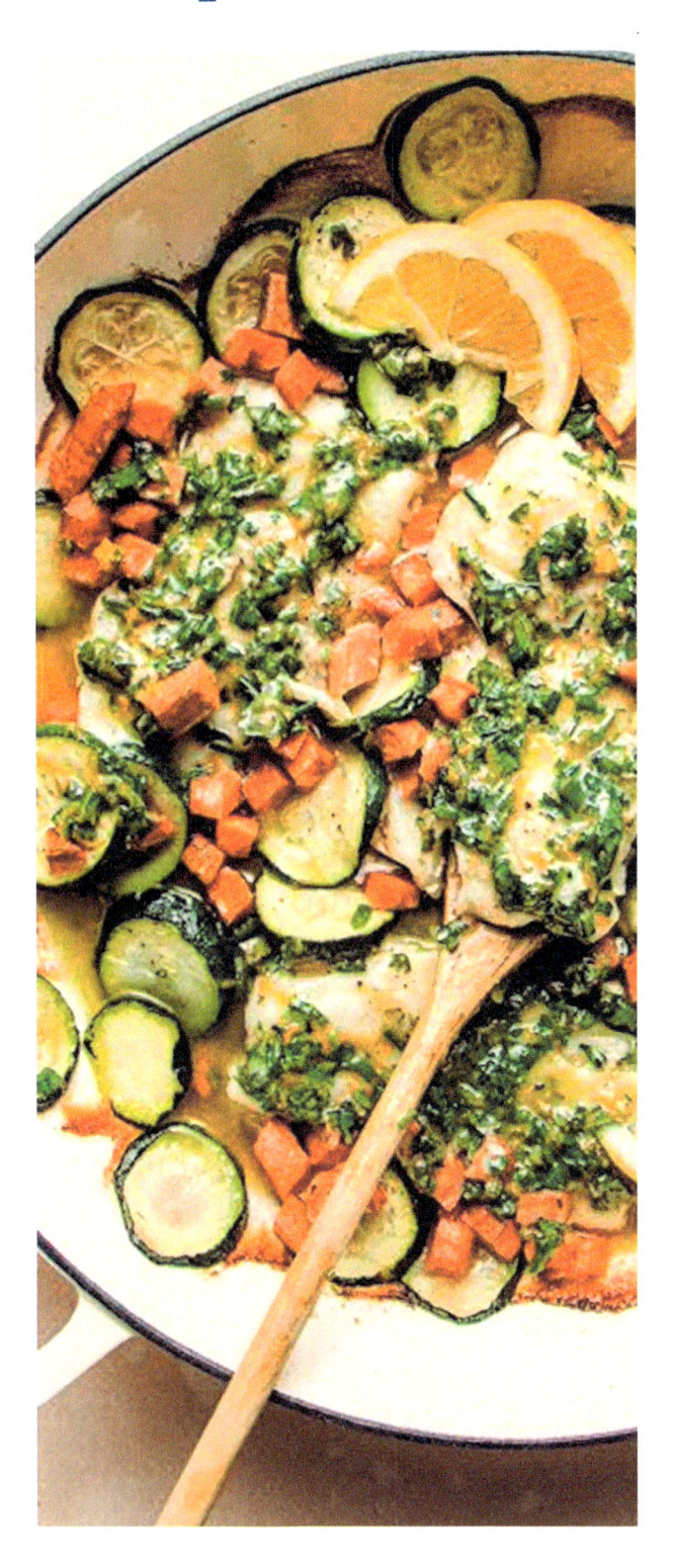

Satisfying Dinners opens the door to a collection of nourishing and flavorful meals designed to bring comfort and balance to your evening table while carefully managing potassium intake.

Dinner is often the heartiest meal of the day, and this chapter offers a variety of dishes that are both satisfying and aligned with a low-potassium lifestyle.

Whether you crave savory poultry, tender fish, or vibrant vegetable medleys, each recipe focuses on maximizing taste and nutrition without compromising dietary restrictions.

These dinners provide ample protein, wholesome carbohydrates, and carefully chosen ingredients to help you enjoy every bite confidently and healthfully.

This chapter aims to inspire delicious endings to your day, making it easier to maintain your dietary goals without sacrificing variety or satisfaction.

Baked Cod with Lemon and Herbs

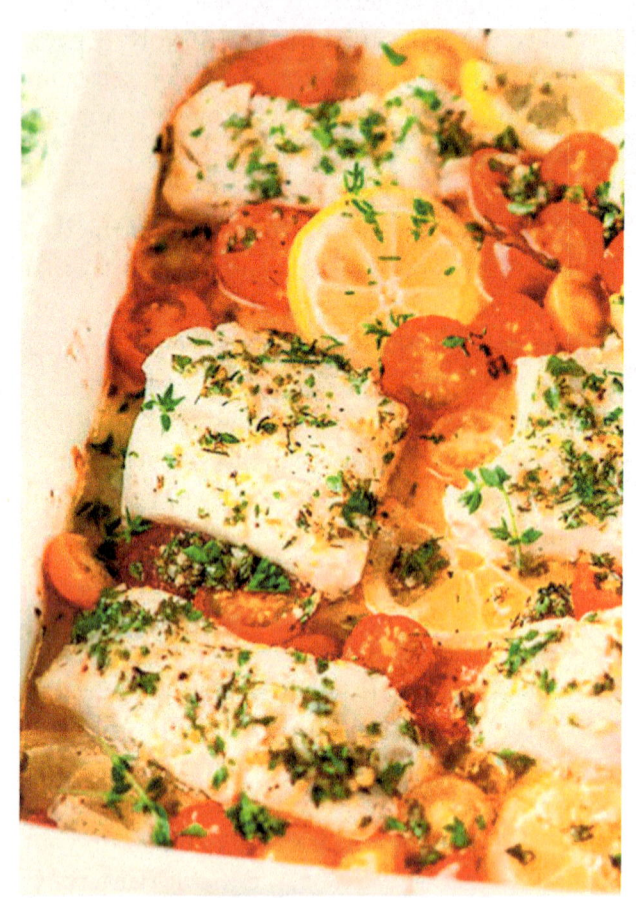

This baked cod dish combines delicate white fish with the fresh brightness of lemon and herbs, creating a light yet flavorful low-potassium dinner. It's simple to prepare, making it perfect for a nutritious meal that supports kidney health and potassium control.

- Preparation Time: 10 minutes
- Cooking Time: 20 minutes
- Serving Size: 2 servings

Ingredients:

- 2 cod fillets (about 6 oz each)
- 1 lemon, thinly sliced
- 2 tbsp olive oil
- 1 tbsp fresh parsley, chopped
- 1 tsp dried thyme
- Salt and pepper to taste

Instructions:

1. Preheat oven to 375°F (190°C).
2. Place cod fillets in a baking dish and drizzle with olive oil.
3. Season with salt, pepper, dried thyme, and chopped parsley.
4. Lay lemon slices over the fillets.
5. Bake in the oven for 18-20 minutes until fish flakes easily with a fork.
6. Remove from oven and serve immediately.

Nutritional Values (Approximate per serving):

- Calories: 220
- Protein: 35g
- Carbohydrates: 2g
- Fat: 7g
- Potassium: 300mg
- Sodium: 150mg
- Fiber: 0g

Cooking Tips:

- Use fresh cod for the best flavor and texture.

- Avoid overbaking to keep the fish moist.

- Fresh herbs add flavor without adding potassium.

Health Benefits:

- Cod is a lean source of protein, low in potassium and ideal for kidney-friendly diets.

- Olive oil provides heart-healthy fats.

- Lemon and herbs enhance flavor while offering antioxidants.

Grilled Pork Chops with Apple Chutney

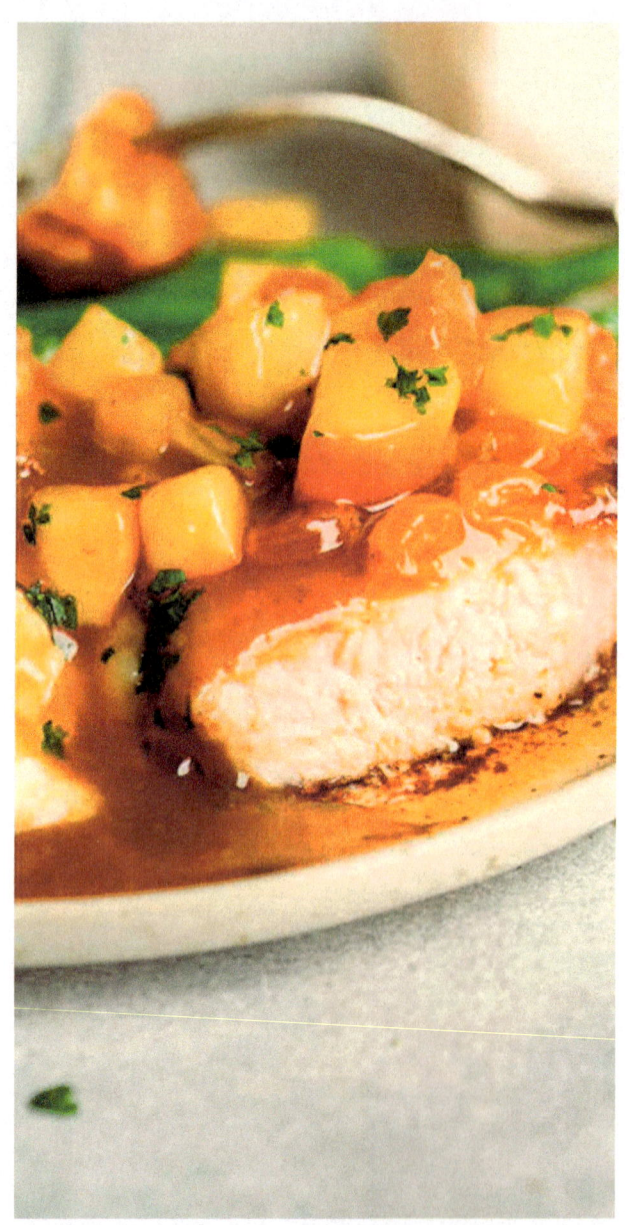

- Preparation Time: 15 minutes
- Cooking Time: 15 minutes
- Serving Size: 2 servings

Ingredients:

- 2 pork chops (about 6 oz each)
- 1 tbsp olive oil
- Salt and pepper to taste
- 1 cup peeled, diced apples (low-potassium variety like Gala)
- 1/4 cup finely chopped onion
- 1 tbsp apple cider vinegar
- 1 tsp honey
- 1/2 tsp ground cinnamon

Instructions:

1. Preheat grill or grill pan over medium-high heat.
2. Brush pork chops with olive oil and season with salt and pepper.
3. Grill pork chops for about 6-7 minutes per side until cooked through.
4. In a small saucepan, combine apples, onion, apple cider vinegar, honey, and cinnamon.
5. Simmer over low heat for 10 minutes, stirring occasionally until apples soften and chutney thickens.

Grilled pork chops paired with a sweet and tangy apple chutney create a satisfying dinner that balances protein and flavors while keeping potassium levels in check. The homemade chutney adds a burst of freshness and natural sweetness without excess potassium.

6. Serve pork chops topped with warm apple chutney.

Nutritional Values (Approximate per serving):

- Calories: 350
- Protein: 38g
- Carbohydrates: 15g
- Fat: 12g
- Potassium: 400mg
- Sodium: 180mg
- Fiber: 3g

Cooking Tips:

- Choose lean pork chops to reduce fat content.

- Peel apples to lower potassium load.

- Adjust sweetness of chutney by varying honey quantity.

Health Benefits:

- Pork provides high-quality protein important for muscle maintenance.

- Apples in chutney add fiber and antioxidants.

- The dish supports heart health with moderate fat content.

Stir-Fried Rice with Mixed Vegetables

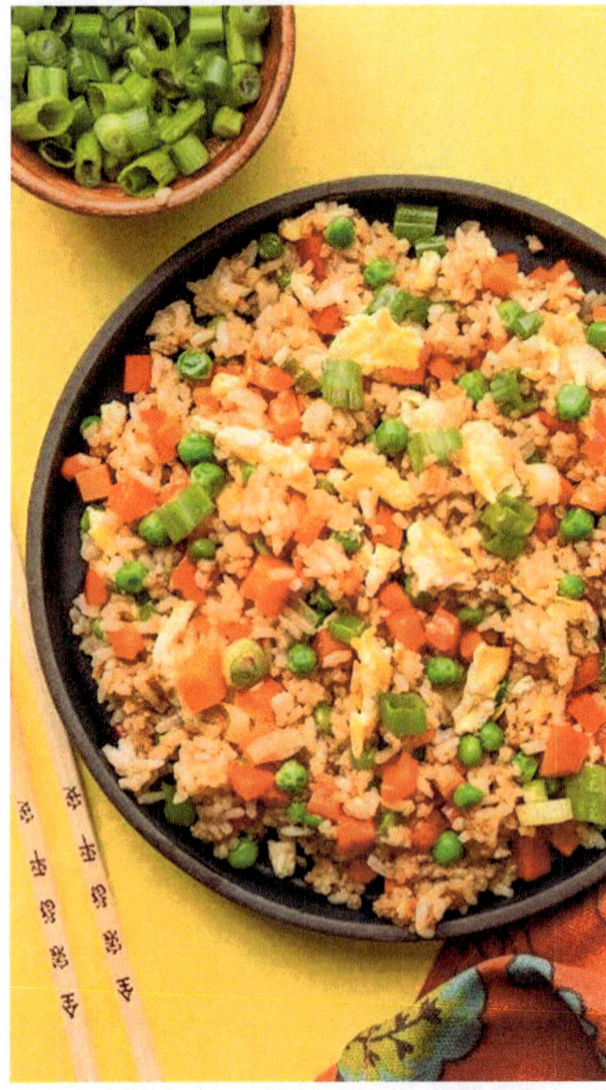

This stir-fried rice with mixed vegetables offers a colorful and wholesome low-potassium dinner that is quick to prepare and full of flavor. Using carefully selected low-potassium vegetables keeps this dish both tasty and kidney-friendly.

- Preparation Time: 10 minutes
- Cooking Time: 15 minutes
- Serving Size: 2 servings

Ingredients:

- 1 cup cooked white rice (preferably day-old)
- 1/2 cup diced carrots
- 1/2 cup diced zucchini
- 1/4 cup green beans, chopped
- 2 tbsp olive oil
- 1 garlic clove, minced
- 2 tbsp low-sodium soy sauce
- Salt and pepper to taste

Instructions:

1. Heat olive oil in a large skillet or wok over medium heat.
2. Add minced garlic and sauté for 1 minute until fragrant.
3. Add carrots, zucchini, and green beans; stir-fry for 5–7 minutes until vegetables are tender-crisp.
4. Add cooked rice and soy sauce, stirring well to combine.
5. Cook for another 3–5 minutes, allowing flavors to meld and rice to heat through.
6. Season with salt and pepper as desired and serve hot.

Nutritional Values (Approximate per serving):

- Calories: 320
- Protein: 6g
- Carbohydrates: 50g
- Fat: 8g
- Potassium: 350mg
- Sodium: 300mg
- Fiber: 5g

Cooking Tips:

- Use day-old rice to prevent clumping.

- Avoid overcooking vegetables to retain texture and nutrients.

- Use low-sodium soy sauce to manage sodium intake.

Health Benefits:

- Provides balanced carbohydrates and fiber for sustained energy.

- Low-potassium vegetables support kidney health.

- Olive oil adds heart-healthy fats to the dish.

Roasted Chicken with Garlic and Rosemary

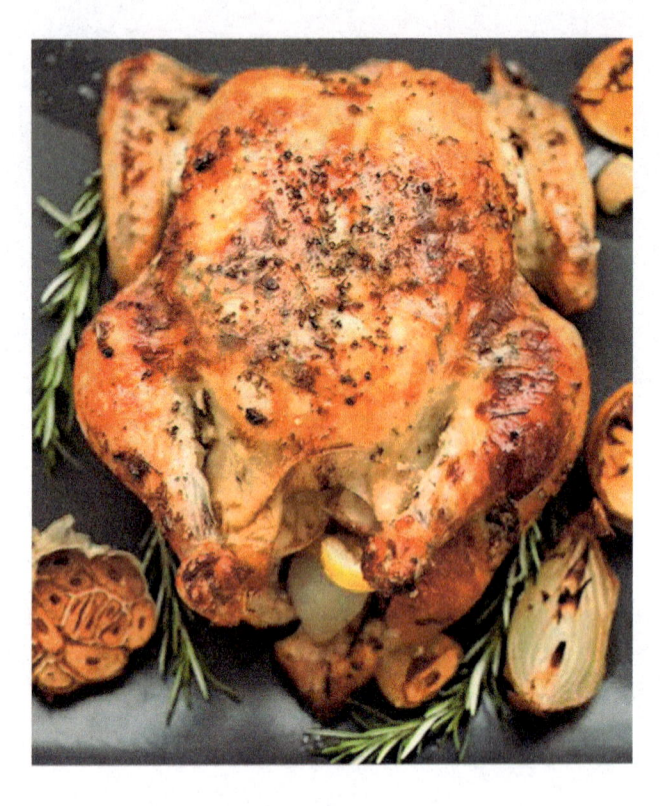

- Preparation Time: 10 minutes
- Cooking Time: 45 minutes
- Serving Size: 2 servings

Ingredients:

- 2 bone-in, skin-on chicken thighs
- 2 tbsp olive oil
- 3 garlic cloves, minced
- 1 tbsp fresh rosemary, chopped
- Salt and pepper to taste

Instructions:

1. Preheat oven to 400°F (200°C).
2. In a small bowl, mix olive oil, minced garlic, rosemary, salt, and pepper.
3. Rub mixture evenly over chicken thighs.
4. Place chicken in a baking dish and roast for 40-45 minutes until skin is crispy and internal temperature reaches 165°F (74°C).
5. Let rest for 5 minutes before serving.

Nutritional Values (Approximate per serving):

- Calories: 370
- Protein: 35g
- Carbohydrates: 0g
- Fat: 25g
- Potassium: 400mg
- Sodium: 160mg
- Fiber: 0g

Cooking Tips:

- Use bone-in thighs for juicier meat.
- Do not overcrowd the baking dish to ensure even cooking.
- Let chicken rest after roasting for better moisture retention.

Health Benefits:

- Chicken thighs provide protein and essential B vitamins.
- Garlic and rosemary add antioxidants and flavor without extra potassium.
- Olive oil supports cardiovascular health with healthy fats.

Beef Stir-Fry with Snow Peas

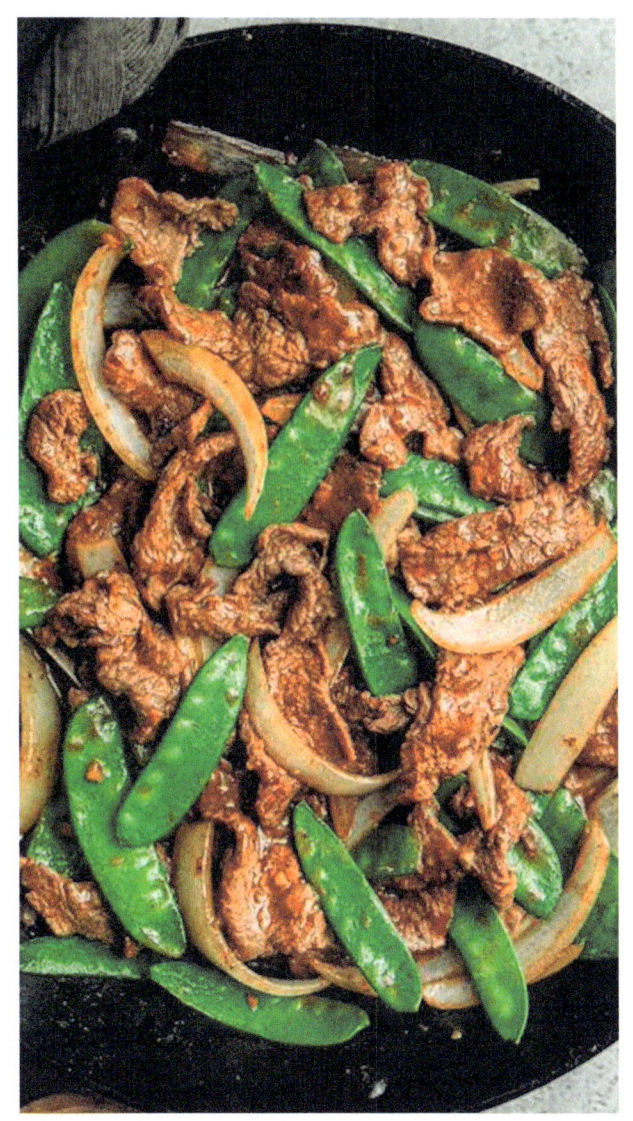

This Beef Stir-Fry with Snow Peas is a quick, flavorful dinner that balances lean protein with crisp vegetables. Designed with potassium control in mind, it uses low-potassium ingredients while packing in vibrant textures and tastes. It's perfect for a weeknight meal that's both hearty and kidney-friendly.

- Preparation Time: 15 minutes
- Cooking Time: 10 minutes
- Serving Size: 2 servings

Ingredients:

- 8 oz lean beef sirloin, thinly sliced
- 1 cup snow peas, trimmed
- 1/2 cup sliced carrots
- 2 tbsp olive oil
- 2 garlic cloves, minced
- 2 tbsp low-sodium soy sauce
- 1 tsp grated fresh ginger
- Salt and pepper to taste

Instructions:

1. Heat 1 tablespoon of olive oil in a large skillet or wok over medium-high heat.
2. Add sliced beef and stir-fry for 3-4 minutes until browned but still tender. Remove beef and set aside.
3. In the same pan, add remaining olive oil, garlic, and ginger; sauté for 1 minute until fragrant.
4. Add snow peas and carrots; stir-fry for 4-5 minutes until vegetables are crisp-tender.
5. Return beef to the pan and add soy sauce, stirring to combine.

6. Cook for another 2 minutes, ensuring everything is well coated and heated through.

7. Season with salt and pepper as needed. Serve hot.

Nutritional Values (Approximate per serving):
- Calories: 350
- Protein: 38g
- Carbohydrates: 10g
- Fat: 15g
- Potassium: 420mg
- Sodium: 350mg
- Fiber: 3g

Cooking Tips:

- Slice beef thinly against the grain for tenderness.

- Avoid overcooking snow peas to retain crunch and nutrients.

- Use fresh ginger to add zest without extra potassium.

Health Benefits:

- Lean beef provides essential iron and protein important for muscle health.

- Snow peas contribute vitamins and antioxidants.

- Ginger has anti-inflammatory properties aiding digestion.

Turkey Meatballs with Low-Potassium Marinara

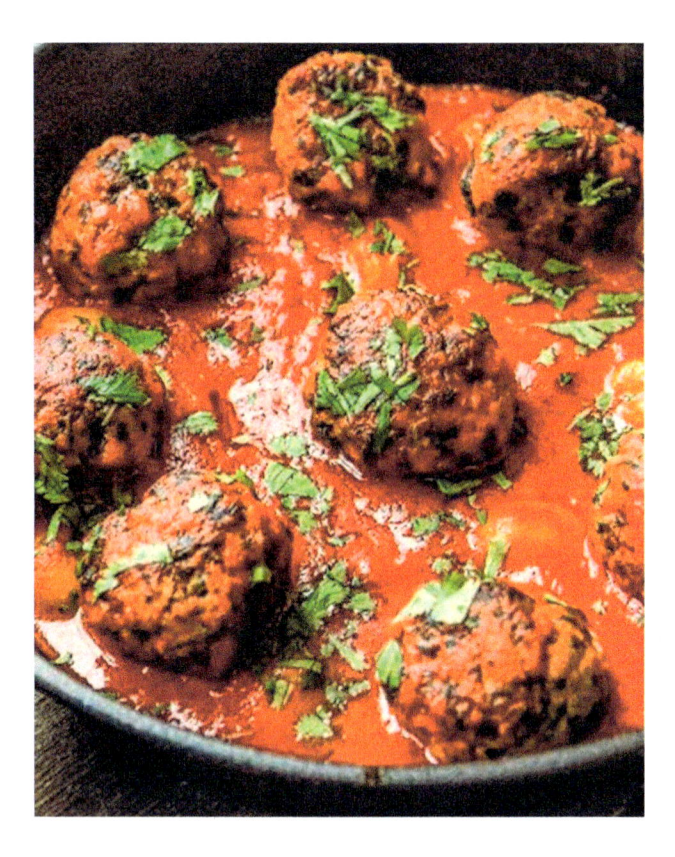

- Preparation Time: 20 minutes
- Cooking Time: 30 minutes
- Serving Size: 4 servings

Ingredients:

- 1 lb ground turkey (lean)
- 1/4 cup gluten-free breadcrumbs
- 1 egg
- 2 garlic cloves, minced
- 1/4 cup chopped fresh basil
- Salt and pepper to taste
- 2 cups low-potassium marinara sauce (made with peeled, deseeded tomatoes or pumpkin puree base)

Instructions:

1. Preheat oven to 375°F (190°C).
2. In a large bowl, combine ground turkey, breadcrumbs, egg, garlic, basil, salt, and pepper.
3. Mix thoroughly and shape into 12 small meatballs.
4. Place meatballs on a baking sheet lined with parchment paper.
5. Bake for 20 minutes until cooked through.
6. Meanwhile, gently heat marinara sauce in a saucepan.
7. Transfer cooked meatballs to the sauce and simmer together for 10 minutes to meld flavors.
8. Serve warm over low-potassium pasta or steamed rice.

Nutritional Values (Approximate per serving):

- Calories: 300
- Protein: 30g
- Carbohydrates: 12g
- Fat: 10g
- Potassium: 400mg
- Sodium: 300mg
- Fiber: 2g

Cooking Tips:

- Use lean turkey to reduce fat content.
- Make marinara sauce from peeled, deseeded tomatoes or substitute with pumpkin puree to lower potassium.
- Avoid over-mixing meat to keep meatballs tender.

Ginger-Honey Glazed Salmon

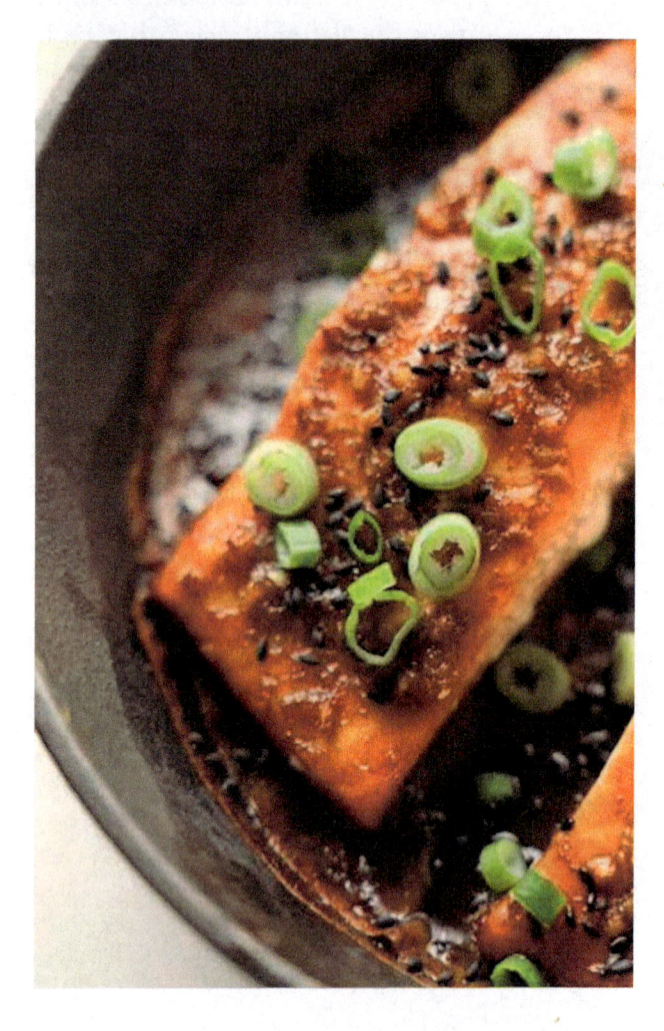

- Preparation Time: 10 minutes
- Cooking Time: 15 minutes
- Serving Size: 2 servings

Ingredients:

- 2 salmon fillets (6 oz each)
- 1 tbsp olive oil
- 1 tbsp honey
- 1 tsp grated fresh ginger
- 1 tsp low-sodium soy sauce
- Salt and pepper to taste

Instructions:

1. Preheat oven to 400°F (200°C).
2. In a small bowl, whisk together honey, ginger, soy sauce, olive oil, salt, and pepper.
3. Place salmon fillets on a baking sheet lined with parchment paper.
4. Brush glaze generously over salmon.
5. Bake for 12–15 minutes until salmon is cooked through and flakes easily.
6. Serve immediately, optionally garnished with fresh herbs.

Nutritional Values (Approximate per serving):

- Calories: 350
- Protein: 34g
- Carbohydrates: 8g
- Fat: 18g
- Potassium: 380mg
- Sodium: 200mg
- Fiber: 0g

Cooking Tips:

- Use fresh ginger for the best flavor and aroma.
- Do not overbake salmon to keep it moist and tender.
- Adjust honey to control sweetness.

Health Benefits:

- Salmon is rich in omega-3 fatty acids, supporting heart and brain health.
- Ginger aids digestion and has anti-inflammatory properties.
- The glaze adds flavor without excess potassium or sodium.

Chicken Stir-Fry with Bok Choy

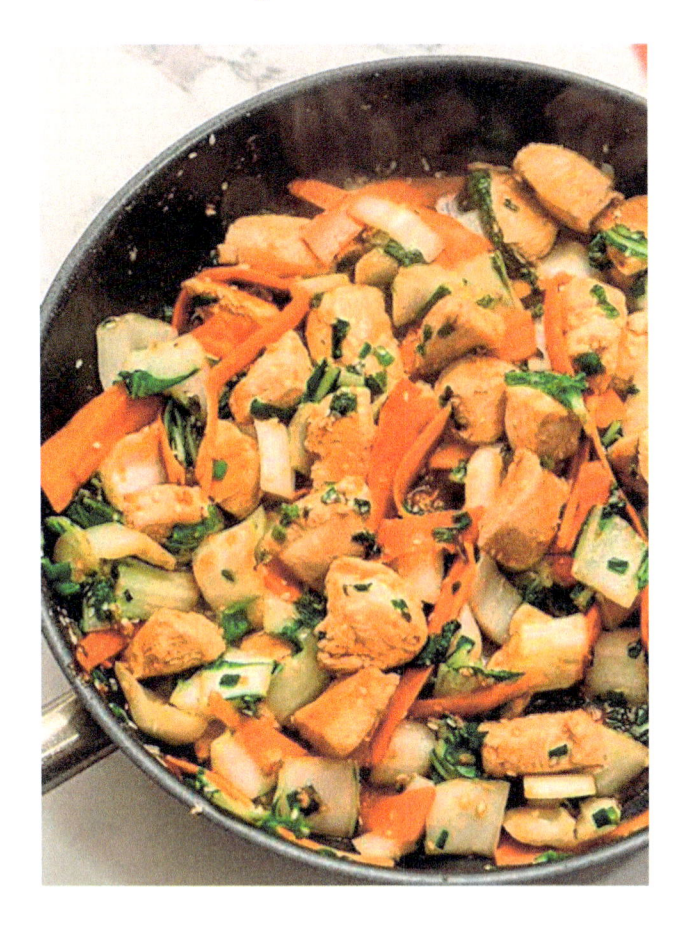

- Preparation Time: 15 minutes
- Cooking Time: 10 minutes
- Serving Size: 2 servings

Ingredients:

- 8 oz boneless, skinless chicken breast, thinly sliced
- 2 cups bok choy, chopped
- 1 tbsp olive oil
- 1 garlic clove, minced
- 1 tsp grated ginger
- 2 tbsp low-sodium soy sauce
- 1 tsp honey
- Salt and pepper to taste

Instructions:

1. Heat olive oil in a large skillet or wok over medium-high heat.
2. Add garlic and ginger; sauté for 1 minute until fragrant.
3. Add chicken slices and stir-fry for 5-6 minutes until cooked through.
4. Add chopped bok choy and cook for 3-4 minutes until wilted but still crisp.
5. Stir in soy sauce and honey, tossing to coat evenly.
6. Season with salt and pepper as needed. Serve immediately.

Nutritional Values (Approximate per serving):

- Calories: 320
- Protein: 38g
- Carbohydrates: 8g
- Fat: 9g
- Potassium: 400mg
- Sodium: 280mg
- Fiber: 2g

Cooking Tips:

- Use fresh bok choy for optimal texture and nutrients.
- Slice chicken thinly to ensure quick and even cooking.
- Adjust honey for preferred sweetness.

Health Benefits:

- Chicken breast provides lean protein critical for muscle repair and energy.
- Bok choy is low in potassium but rich in vitamins A and C.

Baked Ziti with Low-Potassium Cheese

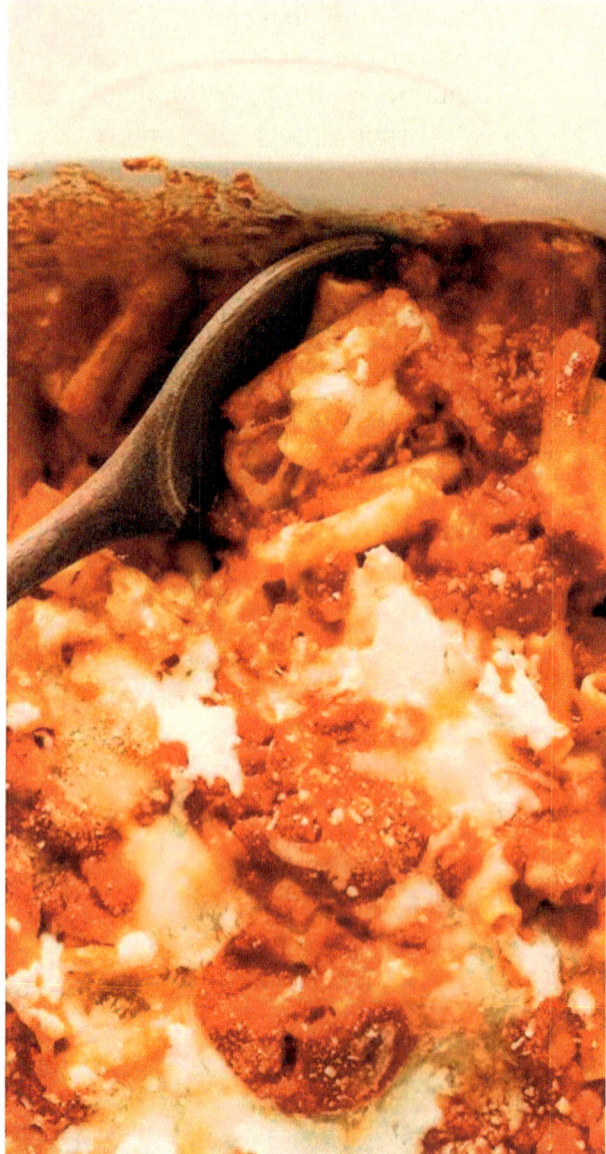

This comforting and satisfying Baked Ziti is designed for those managing potassium levels without compromising on flavor. By using low-potassium cheese alternatives and white pasta, this dish offers a classic Italian experience that is both kidney-friendly and deeply nourishing.

- Preparation Time: 15 minutes
- Cooking Time: 30 minutes
- Serving Size: 4 servings

Ingredients:

- 8 oz ziti pasta (white, unenriched)
- 1 cup low-potassium marinara sauce (tomato-free or peeled/deseeded tomato base)
- 1/2 cup ricotta cheese (low-potassium variety)
- 1/2 cup shredded mozzarella cheese (low-potassium, plant-based or dairy)
- 2 tbsp grated parmesan (optional, low in potassium when used sparingly)
- 1 tbsp olive oil
- 1/2 tsp garlic powder
- 1/2 tsp dried oregano
- 1/4 tsp black pepper
- Fresh basil for garnish (optional)

Instructions:

1. Preheat oven to 375°F (190°C).
2. Cook the ziti pasta in unsalted water according to package directions until al dente. Drain and set aside.
3. In a mixing bowl, combine ricotta cheese, garlic powder, oregano, and black pepper.

4. Add half of the cooked pasta to a lightly oiled baking dish.

5. Spread a layer of ricotta mixture over the pasta, followed by a layer of marinara sauce.

6. Add the remaining pasta and top with mozzarella and a sprinkle of parmesan, if using.

7. Cover with foil and bake for 20 minutes. Remove foil and bake another 10 minutes until cheese is bubbly and golden.

8. Let cool slightly before garnishing with fresh basil and serving.

Nutritional Values (Approximate per serving):
- Calories: 360
- Protein: 18g
- Carbohydrates: 40g
- Fat: 15g
- Potassium: 410mg
- Sodium: 320mg
- Fiber: 2g

Cooking Tips:

- Use peeled and deseeded tomatoes or a pumpkin-based sauce for lower potassium.

- Choose plant-based or lactose-free cheese with low potassium content.

- Avoid adding salt to the pasta water.

Health Benefits:

- Provides balanced macronutrients in a single dish.

- A good source of calcium and protein.

- Comfort food that supports emotional well-being while staying kidney-safe.

Sweet and Sour Chicken with Rice

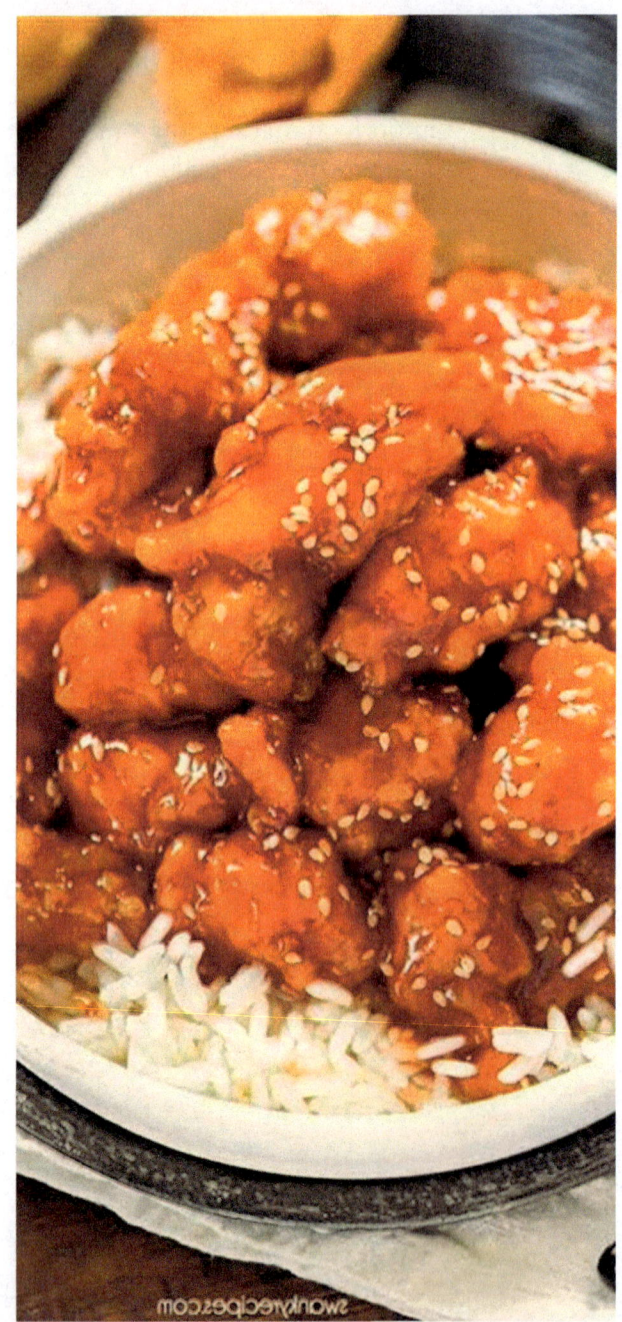

This Sweet and Sour Chicken is a light yet flavorful take on a classic takeout favorite, reimagined to meet the needs of a low-potassium diet. It's vibrant, tangy, slightly sweet, and served over plain white rice for a complete, satisfying dinner.

- Preparation Time: 15 minutes
- Cooking Time: 20 minutes
- Serving Size: 4 servings

Ingredients:

- 1 lb boneless, skinless chicken breast, cubed
- 2 tbsp cornstarch
- 2 tbsp olive oil
- 1/2 cup chopped bell peppers (red and yellow)
- 1/2 cup pineapple chunks in juice, drained
- 1/4 cup white vinegar
- 2 tbsp honey
- 1 tbsp low-sodium soy sauce
- 1/4 cup water
- 2 cups cooked white rice
- Salt and pepper to taste

Instructions:

1. Coat the chicken pieces lightly with cornstarch, seasoning with a small amount of salt and pepper.
2. Heat olive oil in a skillet over medium heat.

3. Cook chicken until browned and cooked through, about 6-8 minutes. Remove and set aside.

4. In the same skillet, sauté bell peppers for 3-4 minutes until slightly tender.

5. In a small bowl, whisk together vinegar, honey, soy sauce, and water. Pour into the skillet.

6. Bring sauce to a gentle boil and add pineapple chunks. Let simmer for 5 minutes.

7. Return chicken to the pan and stir to coat with the sauce. Simmer for another 2-3 minutes until thickened.

8. Serve warm over a bed of plain white rice.

Nutritional Values (Approximate per serving):

- Calories: 410
- Protein: 30g
- Carbohydrates: 45g
- Fat: 14g
- Potassium: 390mg
- Sodium: 280mg
- Fiber: 2g

Cooking Tips:

- Use fresh or canned pineapple in juice (not syrup) to avoid excess sugar.
- Cornstarch helps seal in moisture and gives the sauce a silky texture.
- Stir constantly while simmering to avoid sticking.

Health Benefits:

- Offers lean protein and energy-sustaining carbohydrates.
- Pineapple adds vitamin C and digestive enzymes.
- A great alternative to high-sodium takeout dishes.

Chapter 4: Kidney-Friendly Snacks

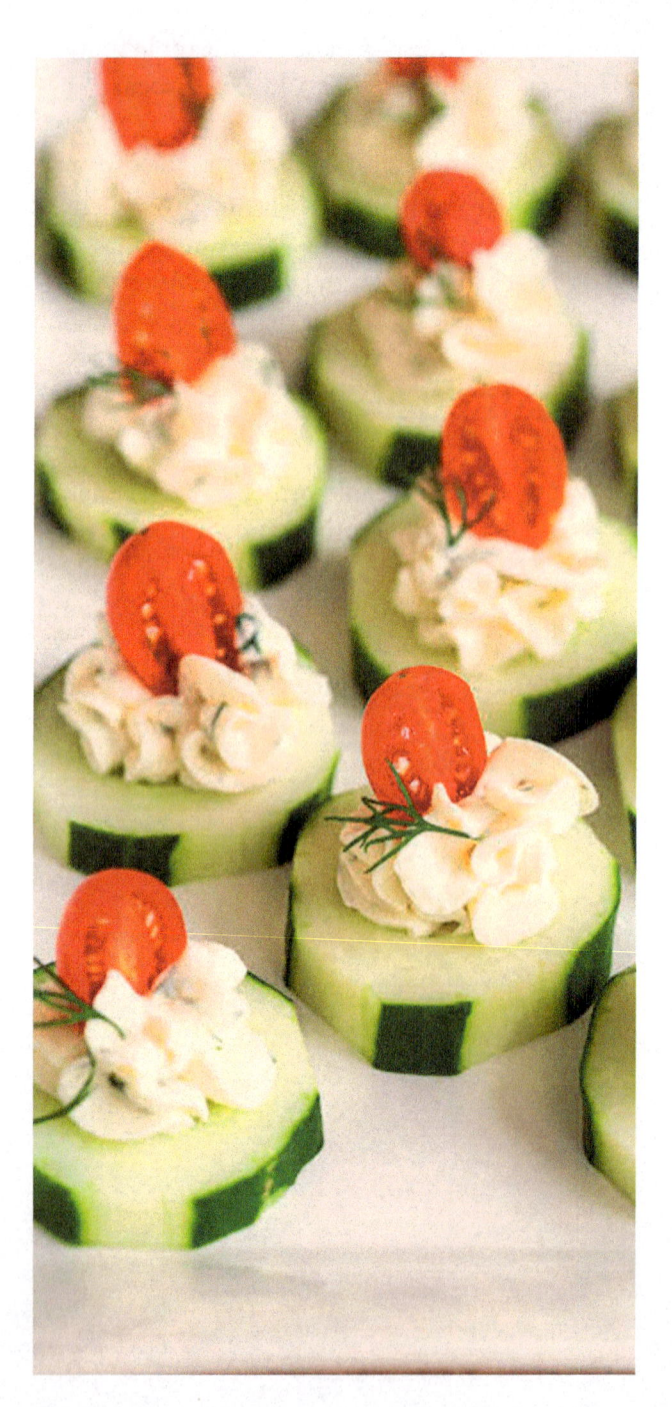

Snacking is more than just filling the gap between meals—it's an opportunity to support your health and maintain stable energy levels throughout the day. In the context of a low-potassium diet, snacks and appetizers must be carefully chosen to ensure they are safe yet satisfying. Chapter 4 of The Balanced Low Potassium Cookbook is dedicated to helping you master the art of snacking with recipes that offer both flavor and peace of mind.

For those living with chronic kidney disease, hyperkalemia, or other potassium-sensitive conditions, unplanned snacking can pose a risk if it includes high-potassium foods like bananas, avocados, or dried fruits. Fortunately, with a little creativity and the right ingredients, you can enjoy an abundance of wholesome snacks that are both kidney-safe and genuinely delicious. This chapter features easy-to-make recipes designed to deliver essential nutrients while staying within daily potassium limits.

Whether you're looking for something crunchy, creamy, savory, or lightly sweet, these snack and appetizer recipes are sure to satisfy. Each option is mindful of sodium and phosphorus levels as well, creating a well-rounded dietary solution for those with renal concerns. From veggie dips and rice cakes to protein-rich spreads and mini sandwiches, this chapter offers both variety and balance.

Cucumber and Cream Cheese Bites

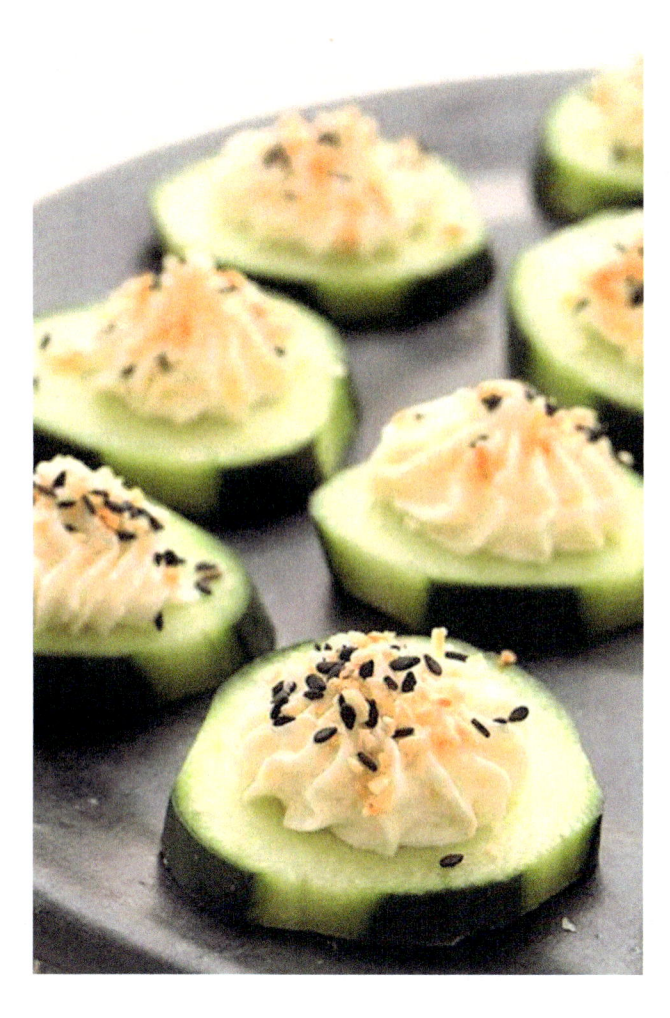

- Preparation Time: 10 minutes
- Cooking Time: 0 minutes
- Serving Size: 4 servings (3-4 bites per serving)

Ingredients:

- 1 large cucumber, peeled and sliced into 1/2-inch rounds
- 1/2 cup low-potassium cream cheese or whipped dairy-free spread
- 1 tbsp chopped fresh dill
- 1/2 tsp garlic powder
- 1 tsp lemon juice
- Salt and black pepper to taste
- Optional: thinly sliced radishes or red bell peppers for garnish

Instructions:

1. Wash and peel the cucumber, then slice into even rounds. Pat dry with a paper towel.
2. In a small bowl, mix cream cheese with lemon juice, garlic powder, dill, salt, and pepper. Whip until smooth.
3. Spoon or pipe about 1 teaspoon of the mixture onto each cucumber round.
4. Top with thin slices of radish or red pepper for added crunch and color if desired.
5. Serve immediately or refrigerate until ready to eat.

Nutritional Values (Approximate per serving):

- Calories: 90
- Protein: 2g
- Carbohydrates: 4g
- Fat: 7g
- Potassium: 120mg
- Sodium: 85mg
- Fiber: 0.8g

Cooking Tips:

- Use whipped cream cheese for easier spreading and a lighter texture.
- For extra flavor, mix in chives or parsley.
- Serve chilled for the best texture and taste.

Rice Cakes with Honey Drizzle

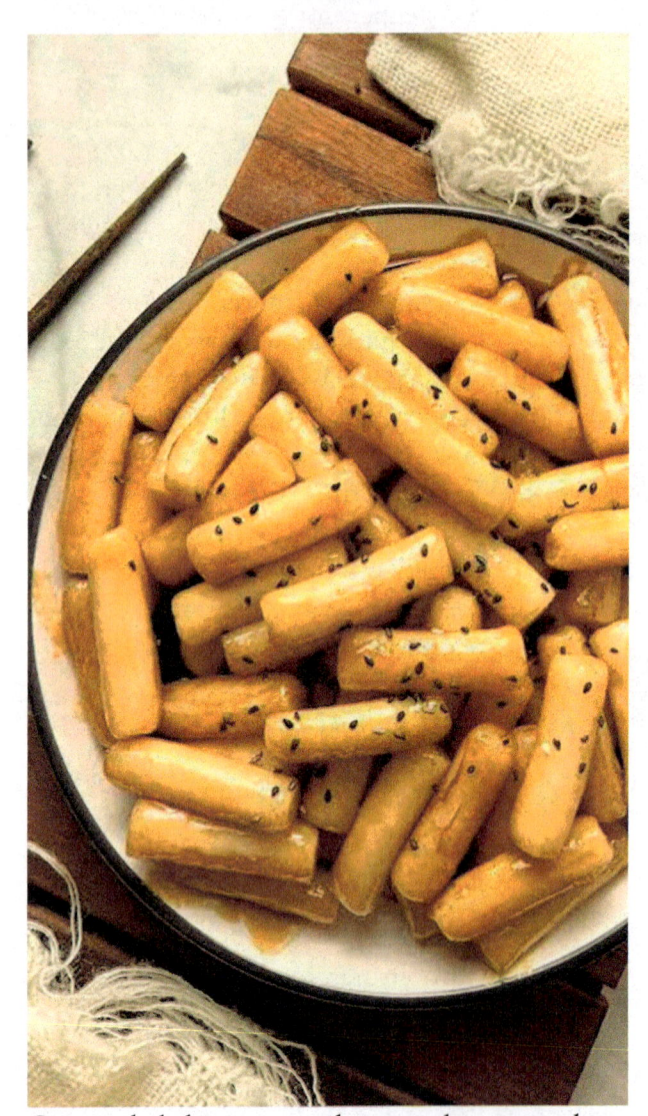

Crispy, lightly sweetened rice cakes topped with a golden honey drizzle offer a simple, kidney-friendly snack that's quick to prepare and naturally gluten-free. This option is perfect for people who crave a light, crunchy treat without risking high potassium levels.

- Preparation Time: 5 minutes
- Cooking Time: 0 minutes
- Serving Size: 2 servings (2 cakes per serving)

Ingredients:

- 4 plain unsalted rice cakes
- 2 tbsp honey
- 1/2 tsp cinnamon (optional)
- 1/2 tsp vanilla extract (optional)

Instructions:

1. Arrange the rice cakes on a clean plate.
2. In a small bowl, mix honey with cinnamon and vanilla if using.
3. Warm the mixture slightly in the microwave (10–15 seconds) to make it easier to drizzle.
4. Spoon the honey mixture over the rice cakes in a thin, even stream.
5. Let sit for a minute to absorb, then serve immediately.

Nutritional Values (Approximate per serving):

- Calories: 120
- Protein: 1g
- Carbohydrates: 27g
- Fat: 0g
- Potassium: 60mg
- Sodium: 0mg
- Fiber: 0.5g

Cooking Tips:

- Use organic honey for richer flavor and added antioxidants.
- Add crushed freeze-dried strawberries or blueberries for color and crunch.
- For variety, swap honey with agave syrup or low-potassium fruit puree.

Unsalted Pretzel Mix

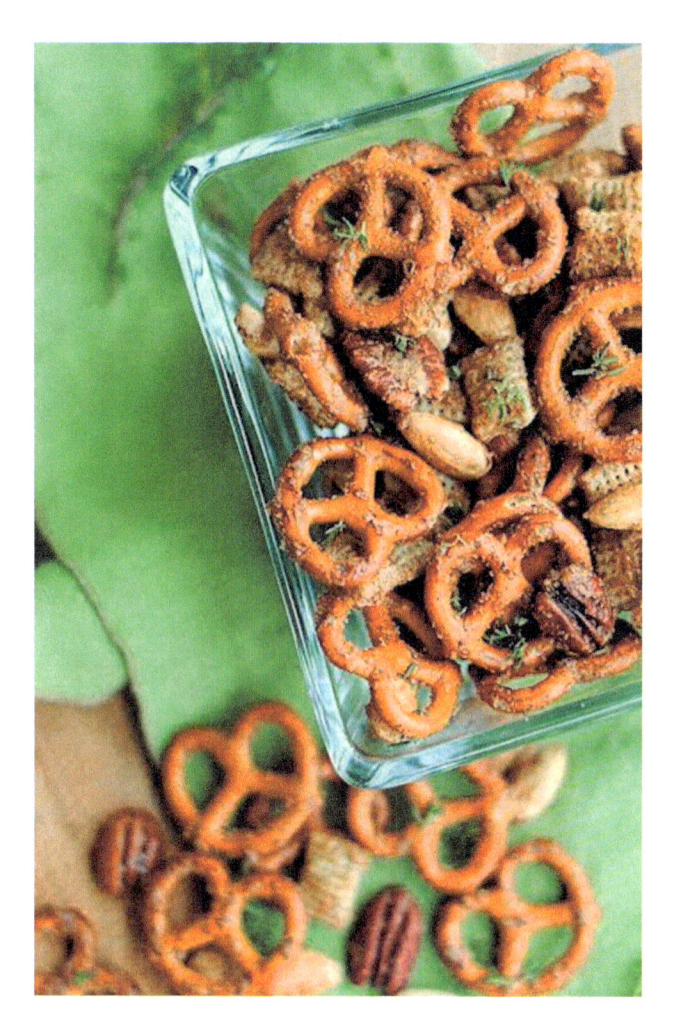

- Preparation Time: 10 minutes
- Cooking Time: 0 minutes
- Serving Size: 4 servings

Ingredients:

- 2 cups unsalted pretzel twists or sticks
- 1/2 cup puffed rice cereal
- 1/4 cup plain rice crackers, broken into pieces
- 1/4 cup unsalted sunflower seeds
- 1 tsp garlic powder
- 1/2 tsp paprika
- 1 tbsp olive oil (optional for coating)

Instructions:

1. In a large bowl, combine pretzels, cereal, crackers, and sunflower seeds.
2. Drizzle with olive oil if using, and toss to coat evenly.
3. Sprinkle garlic powder and paprika, and mix well.
4. Serve immediately or store in an airtight container for up to 5 days.

Nutritional Values (Approximate per serving):

- Calories: 170
- Protein: 4g
- Carbohydrates: 22g
- Fat: 7g
- Potassium: 130mg
- Sodium: 60mg
- Fiber: 1.5g

Cooking Tips:

- Add a pinch of cumin or onion powder for flavor variety.
- Make it spicy with a touch of chili powder or cayenne (if tolerated).
- Store in individual bags for portion control.

Health Benefits:

- Great for travel or on-the-go snacking.
- Rich in whole grains and healthy fats from seeds.
- Keeps sodium and potassium intake low while satisfying cravings.

Apple Slices with Almond Butter

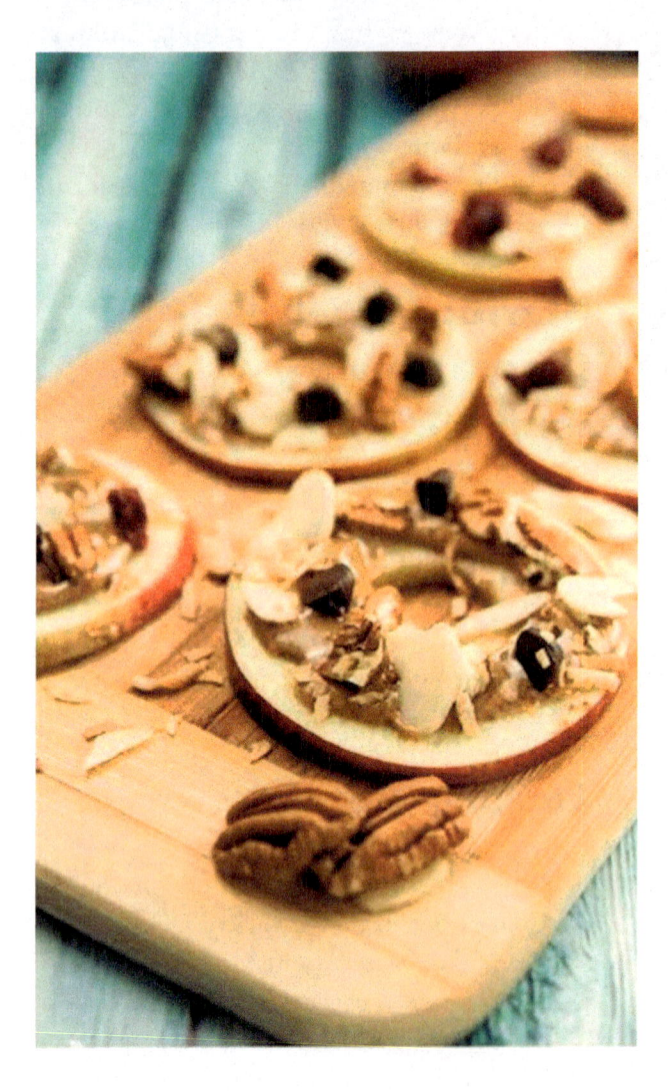

- Preparation Time: 5 minutes
- Cooking Time: 0 minutes
- Serving Size: 2 servings

Ingredients:

- 1 medium Gala or Fuji apple, thinly sliced
- 2 tbsp almond butter (unsalted, smooth)
- Instructions:

- Wash and core the apple, then slice into thin wedges.
- Arrange slices on a plate or small tray.
- Place a small spoonful of almond butter on each slice or serve on the side as a dip.
- Enjoy immediately to prevent browning.

Nutritional Values (Approximate per serving):

- Calories: 180
- Protein: 4g
- Carbohydrates: 20g
- Fat: 10g
- Potassium: 210mg
- Sodium: 2mg
- Fiber: 3g

Cooking Tips:

- Add a sprinkle of cinnamon or a drizzle of honey for extra flavor.
- Soak apple slices briefly in lemon water to prevent browning.
- Use sunflower seed butter as a nut-free alternative.

Health Benefits:

- Apples provide soluble fiber and vitamin C.
- Almond butter adds protein and healthy fats.
- Low in potassium yet satisfying for hunger and energy.

Homemade Popcorn with Herbs

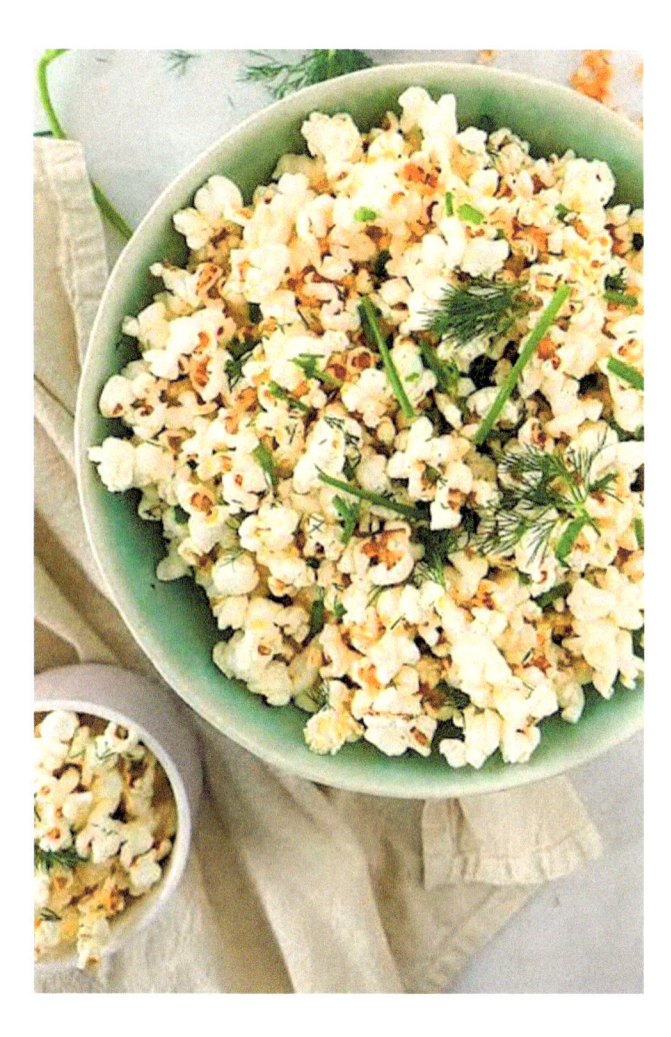

- Preparation Time: 5 minutes
- Cooking Time: 10 minutes
- Serving Size: 3 servings (2 cups per serving)

Ingredients:

- 1/4 cup popcorn kernels
- 1 tbsp olive oil
- 1/2 tsp dried rosemary
- 1/2 tsp garlic powder
- 1/4 tsp onion powder
- Optional: pinch of salt-free herb blend

Instructions:

1. Heat oil in a large pot over medium heat.
2. Add popcorn kernels and cover with a lid, shaking occasionally.
3. When popping slows, remove from heat and let sit until popping stops.
4. Transfer to a large bowl and sprinkle with herbs and seasonings.
5. Toss well and serve warm.

Nutritional Values (Approximate per serving):

- Calories: 110
- Protein: 2g
- Carbohydrates: 12g
- Fat: 6g
- Potassium: 90mg
- Sodium: 10mg
- Fiber: 2g

Cooking Tips:

- Air-pop for an even lighter version.
- Avoid store-bought popcorn with salt, cheese, or caramel coatings.
- Store cooled popcorn in airtight containers for up to 2 days.

Health Benefits:

- Whole grain snack that supports digestion.
- Low in calories and potassium when prepared properly.
- High in antioxidants and heart-healthy oils.

Chapter 5: Desserts and Sweet Treats

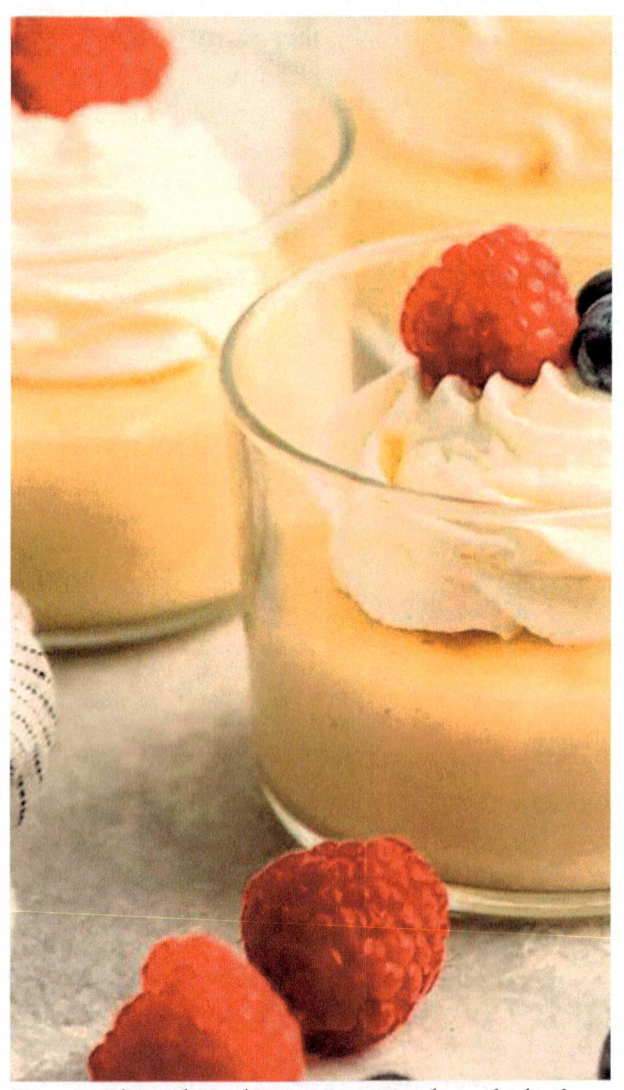

Desserts have long been a universal symbol of comfort, celebration, and joy. But when following a low-potassium diet, enjoying sweet treats can feel like walking a tightrope—one misstep with high-potassium ingredients like bananas, chocolate, or dried fruit could tip the nutritional balance in the wrong direction. Chapter 5 of The Balanced Low Potassium Cookbook brings a refreshing solution: carefully crafted, kidney-safe desserts that allow you to indulge in sweetness without compromising your health.

Living with kidney disease or managing hyperkalemia doesn't mean you must forgo dessert entirely. With the right ingredients and thoughtful preparation, you can enjoy a wide variety of satisfying confections—from fruit-based treats to baked goods and creamy delights—all while keeping potassium intake in check. In this chapter, we spotlight delicious recipes made with low-potassium fruits like apples, berries, pears, and peaches, as well as renal-safe sweeteners such as honey, agave syrup, and maple syrup.

Each dessert is designed to minimize potassium, phosphorus, and sodium, making them suitable not only for those with chronic kidney disease but also for anyone seeking healthier dessert options. These recipes rely on simple substitutions—using rice flour instead of almond flour, coconut milk instead of dairy, and carob as a stand-in for chocolate—to offer textures and flavors that satisfy cravings without exceeding dietary limitations.

Moreover, many of the recipes in this chapter are quick to prepare and require no fancy equipment, making them accessible even for novice home cooks. Whether you're baking a special treat for a holiday, preparing a comforting weeknight dessert, or looking for a make-ahead option to keep in the fridge, you'll find ideas here that suit every need.

Vanilla Pudding with Berries

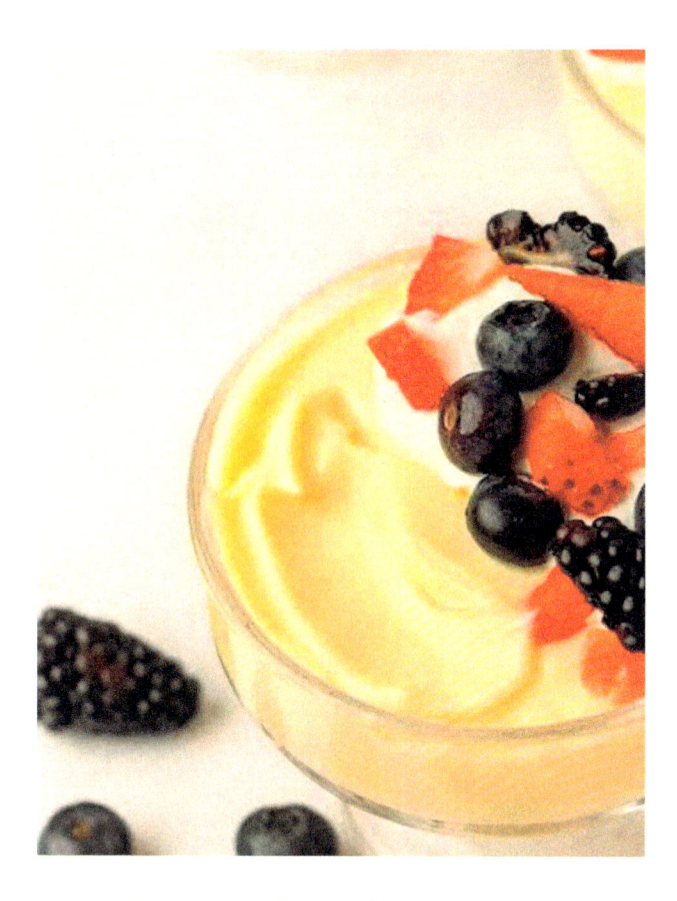

- Preparation Time: 10 minutes
- Cooking Time: 15 minutes + 1 hour chilling
- Serving Size: 4 servings

Ingredients:

- 2 cups rice milk (or other low-potassium plant-based milk)
- 1/4 cup white granulated sugar
- 3 tbsp cornstarch
- 1/4 tsp salt
- 1 tbsp vanilla extract
- 1/2 cup fresh blueberries
- 1/2 cup fresh sliced strawberries

Instructions:

1. In a medium saucepan, whisk together sugar, cornstarch, and salt.
2. Gradually add rice milk while whisking to avoid lumps.
3. Place the saucepan over medium heat and continue whisking until the mixture begins to thicken and bubble, about 10–12 minutes.
4. Once thickened, remove from heat and stir in vanilla extract.
5. Pour the pudding into serving dishes or ramekins and allow to cool slightly.
6. Cover each dish with plastic wrap to prevent a skin from forming and refrigerate for at least 1 hour.
7. Just before serving, top with fresh blueberries and strawberries.
8. Serve chilled for best flavor and texture.

Nutritional Values (Approximate per serving):

- Calories: 140
- Protein: 1g
- Carbohydrates: 28g
- Fat: 2g
- Potassium: 120mg
- Sodium: 90mg
- Fiber: 1g

Cooking Tips:

- Always stir constantly while cooking to prevent the pudding from sticking or burning.
- Rice milk is ideal for kidney diets due to its low potassium and phosphorus content.

Lemon Sorbet

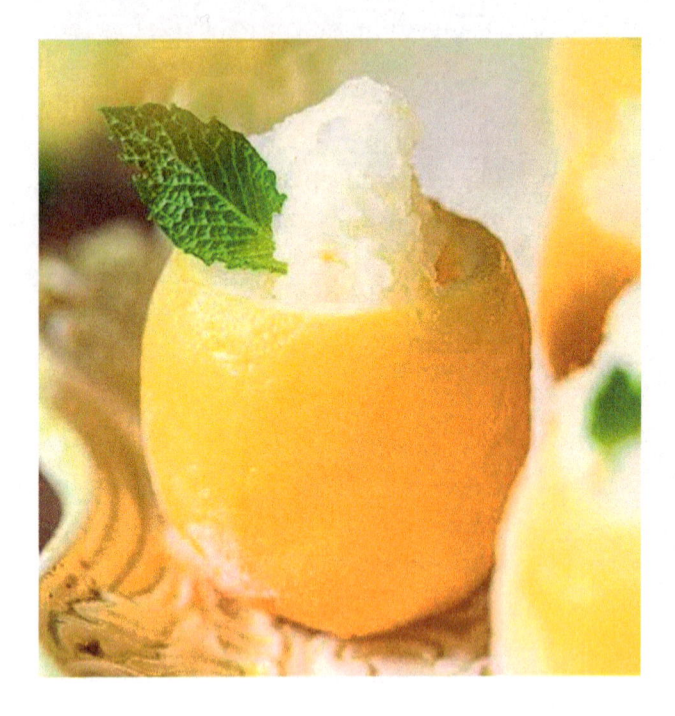

- Preparation Time: 10 minutes
- Cooking Time: 0 minutes (plus freezing time)
- Serving Size: 4 servings

Ingredients:

- 1 cup fresh lemon juice (about 4-6 lemons)
- 1 tbsp lemon zest
- 1/2 cup white sugar
- 2 cups cold water
- Optional: mint leaves for garnish

Instructions:

1. In a small saucepan, combine sugar and 1 cup of water.
2. Heat over medium heat, stirring until the sugar completely dissolves into a clear syrup. Remove from heat and let cool.
3. In a large bowl, mix the lemon juice, zest, and remaining cold water.
4. Stir in the cooled sugar syrup until well combined.
5. Pour the mixture into an ice cream maker and churn according to the manufacturer's instructions until it reaches a soft-serve consistency.
6. Transfer to an airtight container and freeze for at least 3 hours to firm up.
7. Scoop into bowls and garnish with mint leaves before serving.

Nutritional Values (Approximate per serving):

- Calories: 110
- Protein: 0g
- Carbohydrates: 28g
- Fat: 0g
- Potassium: 85mg
- Sodium: 5mg
- Fiber: 0.5g

Cooking Tips:

- If you don't have an ice cream maker, freeze the mixture in a shallow dish, stirring every 30 minutes for 2-3 hours until slushy.
- For a more intense lemon flavor, increase the zest slightly.
- Use filtered water for a clean, pure taste.

Health Benefits:

- Naturally dairy-free and low in potassium.
- Lemon juice aids digestion and provides a vitamin C boost.

Rice Pudding with Cinnamon

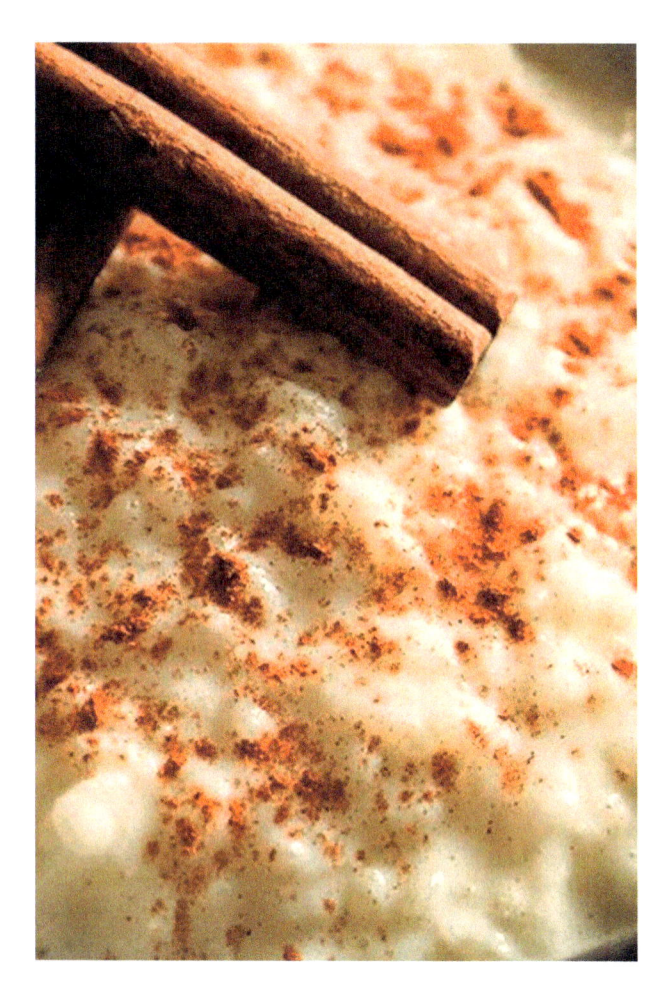

- Preparation Time: 5 minutes
- Cooking Time: 25 minutes
- Serving Size: 4 servings

Ingredients:

- 1/2 cup white rice
- 2 cups water
- 1 1/2 cups rice milk
- 1/4 cup white sugar
- 1/2 tsp cinnamon
- 1/4 tsp salt
- 1 tsp vanilla extract

Instructions:

1. Rinse the rice thoroughly and place in a medium saucepan with 2 cups water.
2. Bring to a boil, then reduce heat and simmer covered until the rice is tender and water is absorbed (about 15 minutes).
3. Add rice milk, sugar, salt, and cinnamon to the cooked rice.
4. Simmer uncovered over low heat for another 10 minutes, stirring often until thick and creamy.
5. Stir in the vanilla extract and let cool slightly before serving warm or refrigerating for a chilled version.
6. Sprinkle extra cinnamon on top before serving if desired.

Nutritional Values (Approximate per serving):

- Calories: 160
- Protein: 2g
- Carbohydrates: 34g
- Fat: 2g
- Potassium: 110mg
- Sodium: 85mg
- Fiber: 0.5g

Cooking Tips:

- For extra richness, use a splash of full-fat coconut milk with the rice milk.
- Sweeten with honey or agave if preferred.
- For texture, use arborio or short-grain rice.

Angel Food Cake with Strawberries

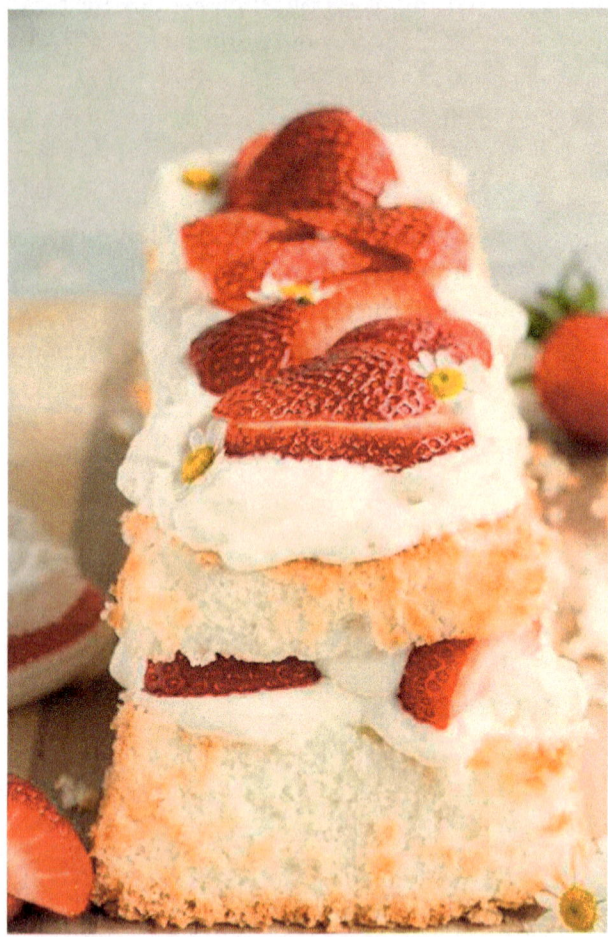

- Preparation Time: 20 minutes
- Cooking Time: 35 minutes
- Serving Size: 8 servings

Ingredients:

- 1 cup cake flour
- 1 1/2 cups egg whites (about 10-12 large eggs)
- 1 1/4 cups white sugar
- 1 tsp cream of tartar
- 1 tsp vanilla extract
- 1 cup sliced fresh strawberries

Instructions:

1. Preheat oven to 350°F (175°C).
2. In a large, clean bowl, beat egg whites and cream of tartar with a mixer until soft peaks form.
3. Gradually add sugar while continuing to beat until stiff peaks form.
4. Gently fold in the sifted flour and vanilla extract, being careful not to deflate the mixture.
5. Pour batter into an ungreased tube pan and smooth the top.
6. Bake for 35 minutes or until the top is golden brown and springs back to the touch.
7. Invert the pan and cool completely before removing the cake.
8. Slice and serve with fresh strawberries.

Nutritional Values (Approximate per serving):

- Calories: 170
- Protein: 5g
- Carbohydrates: 35g
- Fat: 0g
- Potassium: 125mg
- Sodium: 50mg
- Fiber: 1g

Cooking Tips:

- Use a metal tube pan for even cooking and proper rise.
- Avoid overmixing to preserve fluffiness.
- Strawberries should be fresh, not frozen, to minimize potassium leaching.

Low-Potassium Fruit Salad

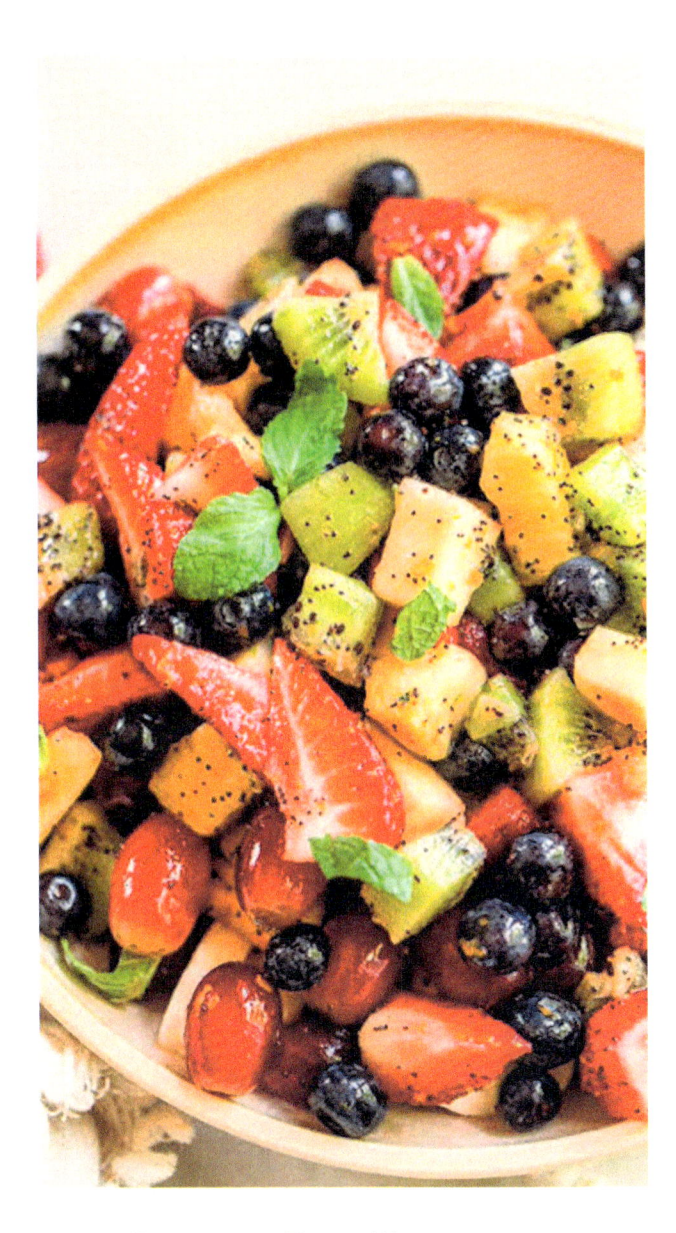

- Preparation Time: 15 minutes
- Cooking Time: 0 minutes
- Serving Size: 4 servings

Ingredients:

- 1 cup diced pears (peeled)
- 1 cup chopped apples (peeled)
- 1/2 cup blueberries
- 1/2 cup strawberries, sliced
- 1/2 cup diced canned peaches (no sugar added, drained)
- 1 tbsp fresh lemon juice
- 1 tsp honey or agave syrup

Instructions:

1. Wash, peel, and chop all fresh fruits into uniform bite-sized pieces.
2. Drain canned peaches thoroughly and dice to match fresh fruit size.
3. In a large bowl, combine all fruit.
4. Drizzle lemon juice and honey over the top and gently toss to coat.
5. Chill for 15 minutes before serving for best flavor and texture.

Nutritional Values (Approximate per serving):

- Calories: 95
- Protein: 1g
- Carbohydrates: 21g
- Fat: 0g
- Potassium: 130mg
- Sodium: 5mg
- Fiber: 2g

Cooking Tips:

- Choose firm, fresh fruits for the best texture.
- Soak apples in lemon water to prevent browning.
- Add a sprinkle of mint or cinnamon for flavor variation.

Chapter 7: 30-Day Meal Plan

Embarking on a low-potassium diet doesn't mean sacrificing flavor, variety, or enjoyment. Chapter 7 provides a complete 30-day meal plan meticulously crafted for individuals managing potassium intake, particularly those living with kidney disease, including chronic kidney disease (CKD), those at risk of hyperkalemia, or recovering from renal interventions. This chapter serves as a practical blueprint, making it easier to incorporate balanced, low-potassium meals into your everyday routine without the need to count or calculate nutrients at every meal.

This comprehensive 30-day plan includes breakfast, lunch, dinner, and a daily snack option to help maintain satiety, energy, and nutritional adequacy throughout the day. Each day is thoughtfully arranged to deliver variety and prevent diet fatigue, with seasonal considerations, weekly themes, and simple preparation methods in mind. The plan cycles through different cuisines and textures, featuring options like light salads, comforting soups, hearty entrees, refreshing smoothies, and indulgent (but kidney-safe) desserts.

The goal of this chapter is to support individuals who are learning to navigate dietary restrictions and those seeking structured guidance in building low-potassium habits. It removes the guesswork from meal planning by aligning with clinical guidelines and renal dietitian recommendations. The plan emphasizes fresh, whole foods that are naturally low in potassium, and many recipes utilize techniques such as leaching and portion control to further reduce potassium content.

Throughout this chapter, meals are carefully curated using ingredients featured in the earlier recipe chapters, ensuring seamless use of recipes already introduced in the book. This way, the reader can refer back to Chapters 1 through 6 for full preparation instructions and nutrition facts while sticking to the plan. Each week includes a shopping list preview and meal prep suggestions, helping readers stay organized, reduce food waste, and make the most of their time in the kitchen.

The 30-day meal plan is also designed with flexibility in mind. Whether you're cooking for one or feeding a household, the meals can be easily doubled or halved. Substitution tips are included to cater to vegetarian preferences, budget-conscious choices, or seasonal availability.

Ultimately, this chapter provides more than a schedule—it offers a lifestyle template, empowering you to thrive on a low-potassium diet with joy, satisfaction, and confidence. By the end of the 30 days, you'll not only have completed a full month of kidney-friendly meals but also developed practical skills, discovered favorite recipes, and found comfort in a structured yet enjoyable approach to low-potassium living.

Week 1: Getting Started

This week is all about easing into the low-potassium lifestyle. The meals are light, comforting, and easy to prepare, featuring familiar ingredients and straightforward techniques. The goal is to help you begin gently while still keeping meals nutritionally balanced and flavorful.

Day 1

- Breakfast: Creamy Rice Porridge with Apples
- Lunch: Turkey and Cucumber Sandwich
- Dinner: Baked Cod with Lemon and Herbs
- Snack: Rice Cakes with Honey Drizzle

Day 2

- Breakfast: Oatmeal with Cinnamon and Pears
- Lunch: Grilled Chicken Salad with Cranberries
- Dinner: Roasted Chicken with Garlic and Rosemary
- Snack: Apple Slices with Almond Butter

Day 3

- Breakfast: Banana-Free Breakfast Muffins
- Lunch: Egg Salad Lettuce Wraps
- Dinner: Stir-Fried Rice with Mixed Vegetables
- Snack: Unsalted Pretzel Mix

Day 4

- Breakfast: Low-Potassium Smoothie Bowl
- Lunch: Quinoa Salad with Roasted Vegetables
- Dinner: Grilled Pork Chops with Apple Chutney
- Snack: Homemade Popcorn with Herbs

Day 5

- Breakfast: Herbed Egg White Omelet
- Lunch: Tuna Salad on White Bread
- Dinner: Sweet and Sour Chicken with Rice
- Snack: Cucumber and Cream Cheese Bites

Day 6

- Breakfast: Blueberry Pancakes with Maple Syrup
- Lunch: Chicken and Apple Slaw Wrap
- Dinner: Turkey Meatballs with Low-Potassium Marinara
- Snack: Low-Potassium Granola Parfait

Day 7

- Breakfast: Applesauce Pancakes with Agave
- Lunch: Couscous Bowl with Zucchini and Carrots
- Dinner: Beef Stir-Fry with Snow Peas
- Snack: Angel Food Cake with Strawberries

Shopping List for Week 1

Produce:

- Apples (5-6)
- Pears (3-4)
- Blueberries (fresh or frozen)
- Cucumber (2)
- Bell peppers (red, green)

- Zucchini (2)
- Carrots (4)
- Lettuce (Romaine or Butter)
- Fresh herbs (parsley, rosemary, basil)
- Garlic (1 bulb)
- Strawberries (fresh or frozen)
- Lemons (2–3)
- Green onions
- Bok choy (optional for stir-fry)
- Snow peas (1 cup)

Proteins:

- Chicken breast (4–5 pieces)
- Ground turkey (1 lb)
- Turkey breast slices (deli-style)
- Eggs (1 dozen)
- Egg whites or carton of liquid egg whites
- Canned tuna (in water)
- Cod fillets (2 pieces)
- Pork chops (2)
- Ground beef (for stir-fry)
- Plain tofu (firm or extra firm)

Grains & Cereals:

- White rice
- Rice cakes (unsalted)
- Oatmeal (rolled oats)
- White bread
- Couscous
- All-purpose flour
- Low-potassium granola
- Low-sodium rice noodles
- White or jasmine rice
- Quinoa
- Dairy & Alternatives:
- Cream cheese (low sodium, if possible)
- Almond butter (unsalted)
- Agave syrup
- Plant-based milk (rice or almond)
- Low-potassium yogurt (plain or vanilla)

Pantry Staples:

- Unsalted popcorn kernels
- Honey
- Maple syrup (pure)
- Olive oil
- Vinegar (apple cider or white)
- Low-sodium soy sauce
- Seasonings (cinnamon, black pepper, onion powder, garlic powder)

Snacks & Miscellaneous:

- Unsalted pretzels
- Vanilla pudding mix (low-potassium)
- Angel food cake mix or pre-made
- Baking powder, baking soda

Week 2: Building Momentum

This week builds on your foundation from Week 1, introducing bolder flavors and slightly more complex textures while maintaining simplicity. You'll find more diverse proteins, creative vegetarian options, and new dessert treats.

Day 8

- Breakfast: Scrambled Tofu with Bell Peppers
- Lunch: Low-Potassium Lentil Soup
- Dinner: Chicken Stir-Fry with Bok Choy
- Snack: Vanilla Pudding with Berries

Day 9

- Breakfast: Rye Toast with Cream Cheese and Strawberries
- Lunch: Grilled Chicken Salad with Cranberries
- Dinner: Ginger-Honey Glazed Salmon
- Snack: Lemon Sorbet

Day 10

- Breakfast: Banana-Free Breakfast Muffins
- Lunch: Quinoa Salad with Roasted Vegetables
- Dinner: Baked Ziti with Low-Potassium Cheese
- Snack: Rice Pudding with Cinnamon

Day 11

- Breakfast: Oatmeal with Cinnamon and Pears
- Lunch: Couscous Bowl with Zucchini and Carrots
- Dinner: Roasted Chicken with Garlic and Rosemary
- Snack: Apple Slices with Almond Butter

Day 12

- Breakfast: Creamy Rice Porridge with Apples
- Lunch: Chicken and Apple Slaw Wrap
- Dinner: Turkey Meatballs with Low-Potassium Marinara
- Snack: Low-Potassium Fruit Salad

Day 13

- Breakfast: Herbed Egg White Omelet
- Lunch: Egg Salad Lettuce Wraps
- Dinner: Stir-Fried Rice with Mixed Vegetables
- Snack: Homemade Popcorn with Herbs

Day 14

- Breakfast: Blueberry Pancakes with Maple Syrup
- Lunch: Tuna Salad on White Bread
- Dinner: Baked Cod with Lemon and Herbs
- Snack: Cucumber and Cream Cheese Bites

Shopping List for Week 2

Produce:

- Bell peppers
- Strawberries
- Blueberries
- Apples
- Pears
- Cucumbers
- Zucchini
- Carrots
- Garlic
- Onions
- Bok choy
- Lemons
- Berries (mixed)
- Fresh herbs (cilantro, parsley, dill)

Proteins:

- Tofu (firm or extra firm)
- Chicken breast

- Ground turkey
- Salmon fillets
- Eggs
- Canned tuna
- Turkey breast slices
- Lentils (pre-cooked or dry)

Grains & Cereals:

- Rye bread
- White bread
- Couscous
- Rice noodles
- White rice
- Oats
- Low-potassium granola
- Pasta (low-protein or white ziti)
- Baking mix for muffins or pancakes

Dairy & Alternatives:

- Cream cheese
- Almond milk
- Plant-based yogurt
- Vanilla pudding
- Rice milk

Snacks & Desserts:

- Sorbet (lemon or berry)
- Angel food cake
- Rice cakes
- Unsalted popcorn
- Vanilla pudding
- Cinnamon

Pantry & Miscellaneous:

- Olive oil
- Honey
- Maple syrup
- Vinegar
- Seasonings (ginger, garlic powder, onion powder, herbs)
- Low-sodium soy sauce
- Low-potassium tomato sauce

Week 3: Exploring New Flavors

This week introduces international flavors, creative ingredient pairings, and new textures. The meals are designed to stimulate the palate while keeping potassium levels in check. Expect dishes inspired by Mediterranean, Asian, and American comfort food traditions.

Day 15

- Breakfast: Low-Potassium Granola Parfait
- Lunch: Stuffed Bell Peppers with Ground Turkey
- Dinner: Chicken Stir-Fry with Bok Choy
- Snack: Angel Food Cake with Strawberries

Day 16

- Breakfast: Scrambled Tofu with Bell Peppers
- Lunch: Rice Noodle Bowl with Fresh Herbs
- Dinner: Grilled Pork Chops with Apple Chutney
- Snack: Unsalted Pretzel Mix

Day 17

- Breakfast: Oatmeal with Cinnamon and Pears

- Lunch: Egg Salad Lettuce Wraps
- Dinner: Sweet and Sour Chicken with Rice
- Snack: Lemon Sorbet

Day 18

- Breakfast: Applesauce Pancakes with Agave
- Lunch: Tuna Salad on White Bread
- Dinner: Turkey Meatballs with Low-Potassium Marinara
- Snack: Homemade Popcorn with Herbs

Day 19

- Breakfast: Creamy Rice Porridge with Apples
- Lunch: Grilled Chicken Salad with Cranberries
- Dinner: Baked Cod with Lemon and Herbs
- Snack: Cucumber and Cream Cheese Bites

Day 20

- Breakfast: Banana-Free Breakfast Muffins
- Lunch: Chicken and Apple Slaw Wrap
- Dinner: Stir-Fried Rice with Mixed Vegetables
- Snack: Vanilla Pudding with Berries

Day 21

- Breakfast: Rye Toast with Cream Cheese and Strawberries
- Lunch: Quinoa Salad with Roasted Vegetables
- Dinner: Beef Stir-Fry with Snow Peas
- Snack: Low-Potassium Fruit Salad

Shopping List for Week 3

Produce:

- Bell peppers
- Apples
- Pears
- Strawberries
- Bok choy
- Snow peas
- Fresh herbs (mint, cilantro, basil)
- Garlic
- Lemons
- Onions
- Carrots
- Zucchini
- Cucumber

Proteins:

- Chicken breast
- Ground turkey
- Pork chops
- Tofu
- Turkey meatballs or ground turkey
- Canned tuna
- Eggs

Grains & Cereals:

- White rice
- Rice noodles
- Oats
- Couscous
- White bread
- Low-potassium granola
- Rye toast

Dairy & Alternatives:

- Cream cheese
- Almond milk
- Yogurt (low-potassium)
- Vanilla pudding mix
- Lemon sorbet

Pantry & Miscellaneous:

- Maple syrup
- Agave syrup
- Olive oil
- Unsalted pretzels
- Popcorn kernels
- Low-sodium soy sauce
- Tomato sauce (low potassium)
- Onion and garlic powder
- Cinnamon
- Vinegar
- Honey

Week 4: Maintaining the Lifestyle

Week 4 focuses on consistency and empowerment—helping you build habits that can continue beyond this 30-day plan. The meals reflect the balance of flavor, nutrition, and ease, reinforcing the idea that a low-potassium diet can be both satisfying and sustainable.

Day 22

- Breakfast: Blueberry Pancakes with Maple Syrup
- Lunch: Couscous Bowl with Zucchini and Carrots
- Dinner: Ginger-Honey Glazed Salmon
- Snack: Apple Slices with Almond Butter

Day 23

- Breakfast: Low-Potassium Smoothie Bowl
- Lunch: Turkey and Cucumber Sandwich
- Dinner: Baked Ziti with Low-Potassium Cheese
- Snack: Lemon Sorbet

Day 24

- Breakfast: Herbed Egg White Omelet
- Lunch: Stuffed Bell Peppers with Ground Turkey
- Dinner: Roasted Chicken with Garlic and Rosemary
- Snack: Cucumber and Cream Cheese Bites

Day 25

- Breakfast: Oatmeal with Cinnamon and Pears
- Lunch: Chicken and Apple Slaw Wrap
- Dinner: Stir-Fried Rice with Mixed Vegetables
- Snack: Vanilla Pudding with Berries

Day 26

- Breakfast: Applesauce Pancakes with Agave
- Lunch: Tuna Salad on White Bread
- Dinner: Beef Stir-Fry with Snow Peas
- Snack: Homemade Popcorn with Herbs

Day 27

- Breakfast: Banana-Free Breakfast Muffins
- Lunch: Egg Salad Lettuce Wraps
- Dinner: Sweet and Sour Chicken with Rice
- Snack: Low-Potassium Fruit Salad

Day 28

- Breakfast: Scrambled Tofu with Bell Peppers
- Lunch: Quinoa Salad with Roasted Vegetables
- Dinner: Baked Cod with Lemon and Herbs
- Snack: Angel Food Cake with Strawberries

Shopping List for Week 4

Produce:

- Zucchini
- Carrots
- Apples
- Pears
- Blueberries
- Cucumber
- Lemons
- Garlic
- Bell peppers
- Strawberries
- Fresh herbs

Proteins:

- Salmon fillets
- Chicken breast
- Ground turkey
- Turkey deli meat
- Eggs
- Canned tuna
- Tofu
- Ground beef or stir-fry strips

Grains & Cereals:

- White rice
- Couscous
- Oats
- White bread
- Pancake mix or flour
- Pasta (white or low-potassium)

Dairy & Alternatives:

- Low-potassium cheese
- Cream cheese
- Almond milk
- Yogurt (unsweetened)
- Vanilla pudding mix
- Sorbet
- Pantry Items:
- Olive oil
- Vinegar
- Agave syrup
- Maple syrup
- Popcorn kernels
- Unsalted pretzels
- Low-potassium marinara or tomato sauce
- Soy sauce (low sodium)
- Cinnamon, ginger, garlic powder

Meal Prep Tips for a Low-Potassium Lifestyle

Successfully managing a low-potassium diet requires more than just knowing which foods to eat—it requires strategic planning, preparation, and consistency. Whether you're navigating kidney disease, hyperkalemia, or simply aiming to reduce potassium intake for health maintenance, meal prep can make the difference between stress and success. These tips are designed to help you save time, reduce waste, and stay in control of your dietary goals, without compromising on taste or nutrition.

1. Plan Your Meals Ahead

Start by mapping out your meals for the week. Use the 30-day meal plan in this book as a framework, or customize it to your preferences. Planning ahead allows you to check potassium content, avoid last-minute high-potassium temptations, and ensure balanced nutrition. Keep track of meal portions, protein sources, and ingredient combinations that work well for you. Consider preparing meals in batches, especially staples like rice, grilled chicken, or low-potassium sauces, and rotating them throughout the week for variety.

2. Build a Master Low-Potassium Grocery List

Having a dedicated shopping list tailored to your dietary needs will streamline your grocery trips. Stock your kitchen with low-potassium staples such as white rice, couscous, apples, berries, carrots, cauliflower, chicken, turkey, and egg whites. Check labels carefully for hidden potassium additives in processed foods. Avoid impulse buys that haven't been vetted for potassium levels. A well-stocked pantry and fridge make healthy eating effortless.

3. Use the "Double Cook" Method

When cooking dinner, prepare double or triple portions so you have leftovers for lunch or future meals. For example, make extra servings of roasted chicken, rice, or baked fish and store in separate containers for grab-and-go lunches or dinners. Label containers with the date, and try to eat refrigerated meals within 3–4 days, or freeze for longer storage.

4. Choose Low-Potassium Ingredients That Last

Buy fresh produce that stays crisp and low in potassium such as apples, pears, cucumbers, and carrots. Consider frozen vegetables like green beans or cauliflower as they're pre-cut, cost-effective, and easy to portion. Freeze cooked grains and proteins in airtight containers to extend their shelf life and reduce cooking time during the week.

5. Use Appropriate Storage Containers

Invest in BPA-free, microwave-safe storage containers that allow for safe reheating and easy transport. Glass containers are a great option because they don't retain odors and can move from fridge to oven. Use smaller containers for individual portions to avoid over-serving and to maintain potassium portion control.

6. Incorporate Low-Potassium Snacks

Prepare a stash of snacks such as homemade popcorn, unsalted pretzels, apple slices, or low-potassium muffins to prevent reaching for potassium-rich alternatives. Portion snacks in advance in resealable bags or small containers so they're ready for work, school, or travel.

7. Be Smart About Cooking Methods

Choose boiling or steaming for vegetables when possible, as these methods can help leach potassium from certain foods like carrots, cauliflower, and zucchini. Discard the cooking water. Avoid broths or stocks that may contain potassium additives. Limit use of sauces or seasonings with added potassium (like potassium chloride salt substitutes), and favor herbs, garlic, lemon, or vinegar for flavor.

8. Keep a Weekly Potassium Log

If you're under medical supervision for hyperkalemia or kidney disease, keep a food journal or potassium log. This helps track your daily intake, identify patterns, and ensure you're not accidentally consuming too much. Apps and spreadsheets can help with this, or simply use a dedicated notebook to jot down meals and ingredients.

9. Freeze Single Portions of Meals

For busy weeks, freeze single-serve portions of low-potassium meals like turkey meatballs, low-potassium soup, or chicken stir-fry. Label containers with meal names and dates. Frozen meals can be a lifesaver on days when cooking isn't possible, helping you stay on track without sacrificing your health.

10. Make Use of Meal Prep Days

Set aside one or two days per week (like Sunday and Wednesday) to cook, prep, and portion out meals. Cook grains in large batches, chop vegetables, grill proteins, and prepare sauces and snacks. Batch cooking reduces time in the kitchen and sets you up for an organized, stress-free week.

11. Educate Your Household

If others in your household are not on the same diet, make sure your meals and containers are clearly labeled to avoid confusion. Educate family members about your dietary needs, and invite them to share some of your meals. Many low-potassium recipes are flavorful and enjoyable for everyone.

12. Use the Freezer for Variety

Keep a rotation of frozen meals and snacks to avoid taste fatigue. You might freeze leftover portions of low-potassium pancakes, cooked quinoa, or fruit compote. Rotate these into your weekly meal plan to keep things interesting.

Meal prepping for a low-potassium lifestyle is more than a time-saving hack—it's a tool for empowerment. With a little planning and practice, you'll be able to enjoy delicious, balanced meals without the anxiety of checking labels or calculating potassium on the fly. It's one of the most practical ways to support your health, stay consistent with dietary goals, and free up more time for the things that matter most.

Conclusion: A Final Note

Embarking on a low-potassium diet is a significant step toward better health and well-being, especially for those managing conditions like kidney disease, hyperkalemia, or other related health challenges. This journey can seem daunting at first, filled with restrictions, label reading, and careful planning. However, as you've discovered throughout The Balanced Low Potassium Cookbook, it is also a path rich with opportunity—opportunities to explore new flavors, rediscover simple meals, and nurture your body with intentional care.

The recipes, meal plans, and tips shared in this book are more than just guidelines—they are tools designed to empower you to take control of your nutrition without sacrificing taste or enjoyment. With patience and persistence, you can build a sustainable eating pattern that supports your health goals and fits seamlessly into your lifestyle.

Remember, the key to success lies in balance and flexibility. It's okay to experiment, to make adjustments based on your personal tastes and needs, and to seek guidance from healthcare professionals along the way. Your body and circumstances are unique, and this cookbook aims to be a flexible companion, offering variety and inspiration that honors your individual journey.

Nutrition is just one pillar of health. Pairing a low-potassium diet with adequate hydration, regular physical activity, stress management, and medical care can amplify your progress. Keep an open mind and be kind to yourself as you navigate this new chapter—there will be days of triumph and days of challenge, but each step brings you closer to a healthier you.

Lastly, consider this book a starting point rather than an endpoint. The culinary world of low-potassium foods is vast and exciting. Use these recipes as a foundation to build your own repertoire, incorporating seasonal produce, culturally meaningful dishes, and your favorite flavors. Share meals with loved ones, celebrate small victories, and remember that food is not just fuel—it is connection, comfort, and joy.

Thank you for trusting this book to guide you. May it inspire you to create meals that nourish your body and delight your senses, empowering you to live fully and vibrantly with confidence in your low-potassium lifestyle.

Here's to your health, your happiness, and every delicious meal ahead.

Printed in Dunstable, United Kingdom